THE TRAILBLAZER'S INSIGHT INTO HOMEOPATHY

88 REMEDIES FOR THE 21ST CENTURY INCLUDING MIASMS, SARCODES, NOSODES, ISOPATHIC REMEDIES & THE BOWEL NOSODES

By Lisa Strbac

LCHE BSc(Hons)

BOOKS BY THE SAME AUTHOR

By Lisa Strbac
LCHE BSc(Hons)

**THE HOMEOPATH IN YOUR HAND: 77 REMEDIES &
HOW TO SELECT THEM USING HOMEOPATHY HEALS℗**

**SCHUESSLER'S TISSUE SALTS REDISCOVERED: THE
21ST CENTURY GUIDE TO SELF-HEALING**

For the two trailblazers who inspire me to become the best version of myself. I love you both deeply.

To the beautiful soul who bravely took on a role to help save the world at her own expense. You taught me more about homeopathy than any book ever could. Your work here is done now - be free and happy, always.

And finally, to my husband, for your unwavering love and support. Without you, this book would never have been written.

I love you all so much.

Contents

Contents

Contents

Contents

Foreword by D. Alec Zeck

As I write this foreword, my wife Kylee is pregnant with our third child - a surprise to us all. We hadn't planned for it, nor had we discussed it. Almost three months ago, as Kylee and I were making breakfast in our kitchen, our son casually announced, "Mom, you're pregnant." And he was right. Kylee was pregnant. How did he know?

A similar experience had occurred two years prior. While visiting my grandparents in Oklahoma, I had a sudden premonition. After dinner, as we drove to a park, I glanced in the rear-view mirror at my Grandpa and turned to Kylee, saying, "I think this is the last time I'll see him." My Grandpa wasn't sick, and there was no indication I wouldn't see him again. Yet, two months later, he passed away unexpectedly. How did I know?

Recently, at an event in Mexico, I witnessed two young children reading blindfolded. I tested the younger blindfolded boy with a random paragraph on my iPhone, covered with a piece of paper as an extra layer. Astonishingly, he read every word flawlessly. How could he, without physical sight?

Modern science, deeply rooted in materialism, struggles to explain such phenomena. Typically, scientist presuppose a physical cause. And when a physical cause can't be found, as is oftentimes the case, they invoke a theoretical submicroscopic particle like a "graviton" or a "virus".

What if modern science, and therefore modern medical science, is totally misguided in its obsession with materialism?

Consider this: it is estimated that human beings perceive only about 0.0035% of the electromagnetic spectrum with our five (primary) senses. What if the remaining 99.9965% holds equally or more significant importance? What if the true causes for these phenomena lie beyond the physical realm?

Foreword by D. Alec Zeck

Could these nonphysical causes be fundamental to human existence? Might they also explain women's menstrual cycles synchronizing, sensing someone's "good vibes", feeling someone's presence behind us, or intuiting that our children are in danger?

Given the failure of scientists to demonstrate that healthy people become sick through exposure to sick individuals' or their bodily fluids, could these nonphysical causes also sometimes explain two or more people becoming sick in the same space with similar symptoms?

What if what we are as human beings is "more than meets the eye"—literally?

What if the non-physical, electromagnetic happenings are the most important consideration for our health, and for reality itself?

Water researchers like Veda Austin, the late Dr. Masaru Emoto and more, have shown water's ability to change its physical structure. When put in proximity to pictures, music, written and spoken words, objects like flowers, and even an individual's thoughts, water will start to reflect its surroundings—and re-arrange itself into an artistic interpretation of its environment.

Veda's work, which involves freezing water in a Petri dish for a specified period of time, has made this seemingly magical-phenomenon visible to the naked eye—observable and replicable for not only scientists, but also anyone with a kitchen.

Given that our bodies are roughly 2/3 water by weight and over 99% water molecularly, is it possible that these same effects apply to the human body? Might our thoughts, feelings, words, and the energetic imprints of things have a direct impact on the water within our bodies?

What if there is an incredibly powerful, ancient-yet-new form of medicine based in all of these questions?

Foreword by D. Alec Zeck

Those of us exploring these foundational questions are on the precipice of a new health story. Homeopathic medicine, which is rooted in these questions, is a fundamental part of that story.

Few people on the Earth deeply understand the problems with modern medicine—the abject failures of the germ-based paradigm, the problems with cell biology, pharmaceuticals, and more—while also possessing a deep, intimate understanding of homeopathy. Lisa Strbac is one of those few people.

I am honored to know Lisa as a friend and grateful to write this foreword. Lisa's work, educating and advocating for homeopathy, will be an instrumental chapter in humanity's new health story, leaving a lasting, beautiful energetic imprint on the hearts and minds of people across the Earth.

D. Alec Zeck

November 2024

D. Alec Zeck is an independent researcher, podcaster, speaker, writer, former Army Captain, husband and father of two young children. He is best known for his popular podcast "The Way Forward with Alec Zeck", which is consistently one of the highest-ranking alternative health podcasts in the world. Alec is the Founder and Chief Storyteller of The Way Forward— an organization focused on educating, empowering, and uniting men and women from all walks of life in pursuit of health, freedom, and coherence— and the producer of the viral educational series The End of Covid. He is also the former Executive Director and Founder of Health Freedom for Humanity. Alec received his B.S. in Systems Engineering from the United States Military Academy at West Point.

You can learn more at www.thewayfwrd.com.

Preface

When I set out to write my first book, 'The Homeopath in Your Hand', my goal was simple: to create the book I wished I'd had when I was starting out in homeopathy. I wanted a resource that would empower people to use homeopathy confidently at home, providing guidance in a clear, accessible format. Since its release, the response has been overwhelming—it's become a go-to for both newcomers and seasoned homeopaths alike, often praised for its simplicity and thoroughness. It filled a gap, bringing all the essentials together in one place, and I'm grateful it has resonated with so many.

We are, in many ways, in a golden age of curiosity about this incredible medicine. People are no longer content with just the basics; they're hungry for more, eager to dive deeper into its profound possibilities. Advanced topics like miasms, detox, the emerging array of newer remedies, sarcodes and nosodes are now capturing people's interest. With this book, I wanted to illuminate these deeper layers, offering insights that go beyond self-prescribing and revealing the true depths of homeopathy.

The inspiration to delve deeper also came from my event in London, 'What If My Body is Brilliant?' It was there that I saw how powerful it is for people to grasp the magic of their own bodies. I hope this book ignites that same realisation in you—that our bodies, in their intricate design, possess an innate wisdom. Understanding the energetic nature of disease and how homeopathy can harmonise with that energy opens doors to healing that are both profound and transformative.

By asking my friend Alec Zeck to write the foreword, I wanted to set the tone for this journey into the unseen forces that shape our health. Homeopathy, at its core, isn't just about treating symptoms; it's about understanding and working with the subtle energies that influence our well-being. I hope that, by the end of this book, you will have gained a deeper insight into this energetic nature of disease and will recognise homeopathy's true potential to heal at levels that transcend the physical.

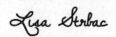

Introduction

Welcome to an exploration of homeopathy that goes beyond the basics. This book is for those trailblazers among you who sense that homeopathy holds a depth and power yet to be fully understood. My first book, 'The Homeopath in Your Hand', offered a foundation for home use, focusing on essential remedies that could bring relief in everyday situations. By addressing symptoms early, we can often prevent deeper chronic conditions that arise from their suppression.

But homeopathy is so much more than acute care. Today, we face unprecedented health challenges: chronic toxin exposure, a mental health crisis and an alarming increase in childhood developmental and behavioural conditions. I've seen the profound impact homeopathy can have on these deep-seated chronic conditions. As awareness around holistic health grows, there is a palpable hunger to understand the full scope of homeopathy. This book was born out of that need.

Together we will explore how homeopathy works not just on physical symptoms but resonates at the very core of our being. While healing at this profound level is ideally guided by a skilled homeopath, the purpose of this book is to offer a deeper insight into what is truly possible with homeopathy—to explore its vast potential to heal, transform and restore balance at the deepest levels, from addressing energy patterns and miasms to navigating the complex terrain of modern health challenges.

This book is divided into sections covering 88 remedies, including those most suited to the 21st century, as well as Miasms, Sarcodes, Nosodes, Isopathic Remedies and the Bowel Nosodes. These remedies resonate with some of the most common energy patterns and symptoms of today.

My hope is that this book will inspire you to see the true depth and power of homeopathy: it is for all the trailblazers who are ready to go beyond—who know that, no matter where we begin, healing is always within reach.

The Homeopathic Renaissance

It's the time of homeopathy! Never has this beautiful healing modality been so needed. In the following pages, I'll share a few words before we dive in more deeply.

The Homeopathic Renaissance

If every home had a homeopathy kit, society's mental and physical health would be transformed.

You might think this is a bold statement, but the potential of homeopathy is profound. Homeopathy, often misunderstood and misrepresented, has a rich history that reveals its true power as a form of medicine that addresses the individual holistically—physically, mentally and emotionally.

Homeopathy was once a cornerstone of Western medicine. In the late 1800s and early 1900s, it was widely practiced, with over 100 homeopathic hospitals, more than 1,000 pharmacies and 22 medical schools in the US alone. This was the original Western medicine, far from a 'new age' concept. Dr. Samuel Hahnemann (1755-1843), the founder of homeopathy, is honoured with a statue in Washington, D.C., the only physician to have such recognition there, reflecting homeopathy's prominence.

However, the publication of the Flexner Report in 1910 dramatically shifted the landscape. Designed to standardise medical training, this report deemed any practices not grounded in the conventional scientific methods of the time to be 'quackery.' As a result, homeopathy and other alternative medicines were sidelined, losing funding and accreditation. Yet, despite these setbacks, homeopathy persisted—because truth always finds a way to resurface.

A notable example of a sceptic turned believer is Dr. Constantine Hering (1800-1880), often called the 'Father of US Homeopathy'. While at medical college, Hering's mentor tasked him with writing an article debunking homeopathy. However, Hering was forced to reconsider his stance when a severe infection in his finger, set to be amputated, was miraculously healed by Arsenicum, a homeopathic remedy. This transformation led him to champion homeopathy—he became an advocate for Hahnemann, and in 1848 founded the first homeopathy school in the world 'The Homeopathic Medical College of Pennsylvania'.

The Homeopathic Renaissance

Hering was not the only sceptic. As a former accountant who trusted the conventional medical system, I began to question the mainstream approach after my daughter's severe autoimmune condition was met with only long-term antibiotics as a solution. A holistic GP introduced me to homeopathy and, for me, witnessing its effects first hand was nothing short of miraculous. What started as scepticism turned into a commitment to learn homeopathy, and it changed my life and my daughter's health.

Homeopathy operates on principles that defy conventional logic. Remedies are not chemical medicines; they are energetic imprints created through a process called potentisation, which dilutes and shakes the original substance to release its energy. The remedies are highly effective and safe for everyone—from newborns to pregnant women—because they stimulate the body's natural healing capacity without toxic side effects or suppression.

Understanding homeopathy's energetic nature opens the door to a new paradigm in medicine, one where we align with the body's self-healing capabilities. As we explore further, we'll delve into the broader scope of homeopathy for chronic illnesses, inherited tendencies, homeoprophylaxis, homeopathic detox and much, much more.

By the end of this book, I hope you'll see how homeopathy is not just another healing modality, but a profound tool for reclaiming health in a way that resonates deeply with the body's wisdom. Whether it's treating acute illnesses at home or understanding the deeper energetic imprints that shape our health, homeopathy offers a bridge to a more vibrant, holistic way of living.

As Mark Twain (1890) said:

'You may honestly feel grateful that homeopathy survived the attempts of the allopaths to destroy it.'

The Energetic Nature of Remedies

It's so important that we appreciate the energetic nature of remedies and how they are made, as explained in this next section. This is because this knowledge has the power to completely reframe the way we think about the material nature of the world we live in.

The Energetic Nature of Homeopathy

Homeopathy serves as a bridge between the material and energetic worlds, harnessing the unseen forces of water and frequency. At its core, a homeopathic remedy is not a chemical substance, but an energetic imprint. My first book, 'The Homeopath in Your Hand', explains how remedies are made, but I've recapped it below to highlight the importance of appreciating remedies' energetic nature.

Homeopathic remedies are made by 'potentising' and 'succussing' the original substance—as illustrated below. This method removes any side effects from the original substance which could be of animal, plant or mineral origin. The succussing process (which means shaking) releases the energy of the substance.

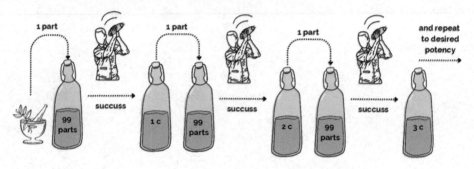

As illustrated above, one part of the original substance is mixed with 99 parts of liquid. This dilution is then succussed (i.e. shaken) to release the energy of the original substance to create a 1c potency (c stands for centesimal scale). Then 1 part of the 1c solution is diluted with another 99 parts of liquid and succussed again to create a 2c potency. This process is repeated until the desired potency is obtained. Remedies in most home kits come in 30c potency, which means it has been through this dilution and succussion process 30 times.

According to chemistry, at dilutions above 12c, no molecules of the original substance remain—a concept defined by Avogadro's number. This is why mainstream science often dismisses homeopathy. However, homeopathy is rooted in principles of physics and energy, rather than the presence of physical molecules.

The Energetic Nature of Homeopathy

Dr. Masaru Emoto's (1943-2014) pioneering research on water molecules offers insight into the potential mechanisms behind homeopathy. Emoto demonstrated that water can respond to intention, words and emotions. His photographs revealed that water exposed to positive words like 'love' and 'wisdom' formed beautiful, intricate crystals, while water exposed to negative words became chaotic and disordered.

More recently, water researcher Veda Austin has explored water's unique properties and its responsiveness to human intention and emotion. Through her method, Austin captures water in its 'state of creation'—the phase between liquid and ice—where it seems to reflect thoughts, words, images and feelings. Her findings suggest that water possesses a form of fluid intelligence, capable of interaction and response. This connects directly with homeopathy, where remedies, prepared in liquid, retain the energetic imprint of the original substance through dilution and succussion. Austin's work visually demonstrates that water can hold and convey information, supporting the idea that homeopathic remedies carry more than just their material components.

Homeopathic remedies resonate with the body's energy fields, gently encouraging the vital force to restore balance. Eileen McKusick's groundbreaking research with tuning forks reveals that our bodies are surrounded by a biofield—an energetic field that holds information about our physical, emotional and mental states, almost like a living archive. Disruptions within this biofield often mirror health issues, yet these imbalances can be harmonised through vibrational techniques. This mirrors homeopathy, where remedies send a subtle energetic signal to the biofield, promoting a return to homeostasis. Through this resonance, the body's vital force is awakened, supporting its inherent ability to heal.

In today's chaotic world, homeopathy brings these energetic principles into practical healing in a form we're familiar with—small, easy-to-take pills that carry profound resonance. This makes homeopathy an accessible, gentle option, especially for families with young children and babies. Homeopathy is a bridge; while remedies come in a physical form, they are energetic in nature, helping us realise the body's amazing capacity to heal itself.

How to Choose Remedies

The next section explores how homeopaths select constitutional remedies, or what we call 'classical prescribing'. It also includes a reminder of how home prescribers (and homeopaths!) can choose a remedy for acute illnesses and first aid situations, which is covered in much more detail in my first book and the appendix of this one.

This section also includes answers to your most frequently asked questions in relation to Classical Homeopathy.

> ## Chronic issues
> Long-standing conditions, such as eczema, asthma, autoimmune issues or persistent mental health disorders, are considered chronic. These issues require constitutional treatment from a homeopath to address deeper, underlying imbalances.

> ## Acute issues
> These are temporary symptoms, such as colds, sore throats, flu symptoms, teething or sprains, that appear suddenly. They can often be managed with self-prescribed remedies and, with the right remedy, tend to resolve quickly.

How to Choose a Remedy - Acutes

This book is not intended to be a self prescribing book for acute health issues - this is all covered in detail in my first book, 'The Homeopath in Your Hand'. However, for the sake of completeness, I've included below a little recap on how to select a remedy for first aid and acute situations using Homeopathy HEALS.©

Remember, homeopathy treats the whole person and we are always treating the individual WITH the disease, not the disease itself. The remedy must fit the symptoms of the individual on an individual basis. Two people may have the same named condition e.g. flu, but their experience of it and their symptoms might be very different—they may need different remedies to match their symptoms. When selecting a remedy, we need to choose at least 3-5 unique symptoms that the patient is experiencing. We can use the Homeopathy HEALS© technique below to help extract symptoms.

Homeopathy HEALS™

The acronym HEALS was created by Lisa to help with remedy selection

 H is for Helps or Hinders - What helps the person feel better and what hinders healing? We can observe what is going on here. e.g. does the person feel better for lying down? or for fresh air? or company? or is the healing hindered by moving about? or warmth/cold? etc.

 E is for Event – What event caused the complaint? Certain remedies have an affinity to certain events (or shocks). e.g. did it come on after being out in a cold dry wind (Aconite)? or after an accident (Arnica)? or after getting feet wet (Pulsatilla)?

 A for Accompanying symptoms– What else is occurring alongside the main complaint? e.g. irritable, snotty nose, fever, thirstlessness.

 L is for Location - Be specific, find out where in the body the complaint is. Where exactly is it and where did it start? Is it the left side? the right side? or does it change?

 S is for Sensations – What exactly does it feel like? e.g. needle, throbbing pain, pain worse for first movement.

As long as the remedy matches the 3-5 Homeopathy HEALS symptoms, it does not matter if you do not fit everything else the remedy covers. Most homeopathic remedies have a HUGE scope of action and can be suitable for many different complaints and states.

Classical Homeopathy

My journey into classical homeopathy began with a single, awe-inspiring moment—a miraculous healing response in my own daughter, triggered by the remedy Proteus. This profound experience opened my eyes to the true nature of healing and health. The reason that this remedy stimulated such a deep healing response was because it was such a great match for her overall constitution at the time.

So how do homeopaths select constitutional remedies (what we also call classical prescribing)?

Classical homeopathy is not just about treating symptoms; it's about understanding the person behind the symptoms. It is a process that respects the individual as a whole rather than treating based on the disease label. Each case is a unique story that unfolds through detailed discussions, revealing layers of health, history and emotion. This homeopathic approach enables us to see the patient in their entirety, considering every aspect of their being—mental, emotional and physical.

The importance of the 'timeline'
A crucial element of the initial conversations between homeopath and patient involves constructing a timeline, a chronological mapping of the patient's major life events alongside their health history. This timeline is not merely a clinical record—it's a narrative of their life journey.

The timeline often shows patterns that link significant emotional events to subsequent physical ailments. For instance, a grief might have preceded the onset of a chronic condition such as Multiple Sclerosis. These connections are pivotal in homeopathy, as these significant life events are often crucial in helping to find the 'right' remedy. Trauma and shock can create a 'disturbance' that leaves an imprint within the individual's energy field, or as Dr. Rajan Sankaran so beautifully put:

> 'The central disturbance comes first and this is followed by changes in the various organ systems depending upon each individual's pathological tendencies. Pathology grows on the central disturbance like a creeper on a stick. What we have to do is remove the central disturbance'

14

Classical Homeopathy

During consultations, conversations are guided by a genuine curiosity about the patient's experience. Homeopaths explore everything from the patient's deepest fears to their daily habits. The initial appointment delves into how the patient handles emotions and stress, significant relationships and pivotal life changes. This exploration helps the homeopath to understand the mental and emotional layers that may contribute to their physical symptoms. The homeopath will also cover physical and general well-being, discussing things like physical routines, dietary habits, sleep patterns, body temperature, environmental preferences and more!

> 66
> Homeopaths treat the person not the disease. Disease starts from disturbances in the vital energy and then appear as physical symptoms of disease
> 99

Hierarchy of symptoms
Once the case has been taken in full, the homeopath extracts the symptoms that they feel encapsulate the 'essence' or 'energy' of the case. In total, they generally look for around 8 symptoms in the following order of importance:

1st - Spiritual, mental and emotional symptoms
We want to select around 5 spiritual, emotional or mental symptoms. For example, mood, dreams, desires, fears etc. As mentioned previously, we are also especially interested in what was happening around the time the person got sick - was there a major life event, conflict or trauma?

2nd - Physical general symptoms
We want to select around 2 symptoms that relate to the whole person. For example, symptoms such as body temperature, food preferences, cravings, sleep. menses etc.

3rd - Physical specifics and disease symptoms
These are symptoms pertaining to parts of the person or the actual disease state, e.g. headache, runny nose, eczema, hayfever etc. We want to select around 1-2 symptoms. Ironically, it is often these symptoms that bring the patient to a homeopathy appointment and yet they are of least importance in finding the best matched remedy.

Classical Homeopathy

> ❝
> 'briefly, in every individual case of disease the totality of the symptoms must be the physician's only concern, the only object of his attention, the only thing to be removed by his intervention in order to cure, i.e. to transform the disease into health.'
> Hahnemann - Organon
> ❞

The final 8 symptoms (what we call 'rubrics' in homeopathy) are cross-referenced to a homeopathic **Repertory** - we call this process 'repertorisation.' A Repertory is a homeopathic reference book containing thousands of symptoms and those remedies that have been found to cure each symptom.

The top scoring remedies are then carefully analysed by the homeopath via the **Materia Medica** (a reference book containing all remedies and their profiles). The remedy with the best overall energetic match is selected—not necessarily the top scoring! It's crucial that the chosen remedy aligns with the patient's mental and emotional state, as these are often the underlying causes of illness. When clear mental or emotional symptoms are present, they take precedence in guiding remedy selection.

We know that chronic issues are those that are unable to resolve on their own due to a deep imbalance of the vital force. Do not underestimate the power of emotions, shock and trauma to create energetic disturbances and imbalances within the body. This is acknowledged by other 'alternative' approaches to health such as German New Medicine, which says diseases are not random, but instead arise from unexpected, traumatic and highly stressful events that the individual experiences on a psychological level. These events lead to specific changes in the brain that are linked to specific physical symptoms and disease patterns.

This is where homeopathy is so powerful, because remedies can touch our spirit and mind, helping to make the unconscious conscious. When we take these remedies they can help move us through trapped or suppressed emotions, restoring health on all levels.

Classical Homeopathy

What if the patient is closed and won't share any mental or emotional symptoms?
This is a question that I get asked a lot and this in itself is a symptom. The homeopath can repertorise the fact that the patient is closed or reserved and most likely the best matching remedy, which will come through repertorisation, will be one that reflects the energy pattern of 'closedness'. It is amazing how, once the patient has taken this remedy, they will be willing to open up at the follow up appointment.

I'm not a homeopath, can I self-prescribe a constitutional remedy for myself or my family?
Prescribing is complex and best guided by a professional homeopath who can deeply assess individual symptoms, emotional states and overall health. Self-prescribing often misses the subtleties needed for a successful match.

Constitutional remedies can also bring up old, suppressed symptoms that need careful monitoring. A trained homeopath knows how to adjust the remedy, manage responses and guide gentle healing. Without this expertise, natural healing reactions can be misunderstood, leading to confusion or even abandoning homeopathy altogether.

That said, for acute ailments such as colds, flu, sore throats, teething, etc., it's perfectly fine to self-prescribe. See the appendix on page 207 for dosing guidelines for acute issues. However, for long-term, deeper healing, always consult a homeopath to avoid complicating your case or missing the nuances essential to constitutional remedies.

I've been working with a homeopath for a long time but not seeing any improvement. Should I change homeopaths?
Not necessarily. Discuss your concerns openly with your homeopath. Sometimes, healing takes time or adjustments and a discussion and perseverance can help. However, If you feel unheard or uncomfortable, it might be worth considering a second opinion or another homeopath who resonates with you.

Classical Homeopathy FAQ

Can my constitutional remedy change over time?
Yes, your constitutional remedy can change as your state of health, life circumstances and emotional well-being evolve. A remedy that worked in the past might need adjustment if new symptoms or changes in life occur. Furthermore, very often homeopathy involves 'peeling back layers' before the individual's true underlying constitution is revealed.

How often should I take my constitutional remedy?
The frequency depends on individual needs and circumstances. Some may need a daily dose, while others may require it weekly or even less frequently. Always follow your homeopath's guidance.

What if I feel worse after taking my constitutional remedy?
This may be a healing response or a 'return of old symptoms' indicating that the remedy is working. Communicate with your homeopath about any changes, as they can guide whether to continue, adjust or pause the remedy.

Can my constitutional remedy address all my health issues?
A well-selected constitutional remedy can support overall well-being and help address a range of symptoms, but it may not cover every specific issue. Sometimes, additional remedies or different approaches are needed to address acute or specific conditions.

Can I use my constitutional remedy during an acute illness, like a cold or flu?
It depends. Sometimes the constitutional remedy will help, but in acute situations, a different remedy may be needed to address specific symptoms. Sometimes what we perceive to be an acute illness is actually a healing or detox response, or a return of old symptoms, so it is best to consult your homeopath for personalised advice.

Can a constitutional remedy help with mental and emotional issues as well as physical ones?
Absolutely. Constitutional remedies are designed to address the whole person—mind, body and spirit. They can help bring balance to mental and emotional states, such as anxiety, grief or depression, as well as physical symptoms.

Classical Homeopathy

Why do different homeopaths sometimes suggest different constitutional remedies for the same person?
Homeopathy is both an art and a science. Different homeopaths may perceive different aspects of a person's state or use different methodologies, leading to variations in remedy selection. There is often more than one suitable approach.

Can I take other medications while on a constitutional remedy?
Yes, but it's essential to inform your homeopath about medications that you're taking, as they may create a 'drug layer' (discussed later) that might influence the remedy's action.

How long does it typically take to see results from a constitutional remedy?
It varies widely depending on the individual, their condition and how long they've been unwell. Some may notice changes within days, while others may take weeks or months to see significant improvement. Trust the process, but communicate regularly with your homeopath.

How do I know if my constitutional remedy is working?
Signs of improvement can vary; they may be subtle shifts in energy, mood, sleep or digestion before physical symptoms change. True healing often starts from within and radiates outward, so be patient and observant of any small, positive changes.

How do I know when I no longer need my constitutional remedy?
When you experience a sustained improvement in your symptoms and overall well-being, your homeopath may decide it's time to stop or change the remedy. Healing is dynamic, and the need for a remedy can evolve. Regular follow-ups with your homeopath are essential to assess progress and adjust the treatment plan accordingly.

Potency

The next section explores potency, including:
- which potency
- extra help with selecting potency
- your frequently asked questions

Potency - Which Potency?

Potency seems to be the area that confuses people the most! Read on....

What potency should I give for an acute illness?
For acute issues you can't really go wrong with a 30c. As I explain in my first book, 'The Homeopath in Your Hand', 30c is a beautiful bridge between mental and physical issues. I can't recall ever seeing any aggravations using a 30c potency in acute or first aid situations.

I do find 200c to be helpful in SOME acute situations. I liken the 200c potency to being like the proverbial 'slap around the face.' When someone needs a short, sharp shock and a very loud message to be sent to their vital force then 200c can be the potency to do this job. So think of an intense burning fever, or an excruciating toothache, or a first aid injury, or intense childbirth pains...then, in these instances, a 200c can be the most appropriate potency. However, even in these intense situations, a 30c will still be effective, it just might need repeating more often.

Lower (under 30c) potencies are traditionally thought to work more on physical issues and higher (over 30c) potencies work on the mental and emotional realm. When would I go lower than a 30c? When the issue is extremely physical and where the healing process is typically over weeks, such as a broken bone, then I might use a 6c. I might also use a lower potency if the individual is extremely sensitive, such as a 12c or 15c (and personally I find 15c to be a bit more gentle than a 12c).

Ok, so what potency for chronic or long term illnesses?
Individuals should ideally see a homeopath for chronic issues. Even homeopaths see homeopaths because it is VERY hard to see oneself objectively. In classical homeopathy, potency selection is always individualised. While some people's vital force wants a 10m repeated frequently, other's find profound healing with just a one-off 30c. Yes, even a 30c can trigger deep healing in chronic issues—in fact, I've witnessed this even with a 12c. Generally we want to select a potency that MATCHES the vitality and energy of the patient. Once we get into really high potencies (such as a 50m) they even have the power to impact the individuals around us.

Remedies FAQs

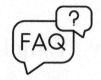

Is higher potency always better?
No, the best potency depends on the individual and their specific condition. Higher potencies like 200c or 1m can be more intense, while lower potencies like 6c or 30c may be gentler and suitable for more sensitive individuals, but this is not always the case! It is always about treating the individual and matching the potency to their energy.

How do I know when a potency is too high?
Signs like strong aggravations (an initial worsening of symptoms) or feeling overly emotional or restless might suggest the potency was too high.

Why are there so many potencies available for a single remedy?
Different potencies target different levels of the body and mind. The wide range of potencies allows homeopaths to tailor treatment specifically to the needs of each patient, making the remedy more effective.

I felt so good on my remedy; why can't I keep taking it?
Homeopathy follows the principle of the minimum dose—using the smallest amount of a remedy needed to stimulate the body's healing response. Repeated doses of a well-matched remedy, especially when not needed, can disrupt the healing process with a risk that the individual may prove the remedy (see page 26 for more information on provings). Once improvement is noted, it's best to stop taking the remedy and only repeat if symptoms return.

What is the most important thing to remember when choosing a potency?
Always match the remedy's potency to the sensitivity and current state of the person receiving it. A remedy is most effective when it resonates with the individual's energy, regardless of the numerical potency. Always start low if unsure and consult a homeopath for guidance.

Remedies FAQs

What are homochords?
Homochords are homeopathic preparations containing multiple potencies of the same remedy, often ranging from low to high. Some say that this combination is intended to cover a broader range of action and address different layers of symptoms or stages of illness in a patient.

What are Fibonacci potencies?
Fibonacci potencies are a way of using homeopathic remedies based on a natural sequence of numbers (1, 2, 3, 5, 8, 13, 21, 34 and so on). This sequence is found throughout nature, like in the arrangement of leaves or the pattern of a sunflower's seeds. In homeopathy, remedies are given in potencies that follow these steps (so 1c, 2c, 3c, 5c, 8c, 13c, 21c, 34c and so on), with the idea that this approach may align more naturally with the body's own rhythms and healing processes, potentially enhancing the effectiveness of the remedy.

Is it placebo? Or just due to intention?
No, homeopathy is not merely a placebo or based on intention alone. Numerous clinical studies have shown homeopathy's effectiveness beyond the placebo effect. A meta-analysis by Linde et al (1997), published in The Lancet, reviewed 89 placebo-controlled trials of homeopathy and concluded that homeopathy is more effective than a placebo. While the authors also noted the need for higher quality trials, the results suggest a significant effect of homeopathy beyond mere placebo.

If homeopathy were simply due to intention, it wouldn't explain the countless cases where animals, plants and babies—who have no concept of treatment or expectation—respond positively to homeopathic remedies. Nor could it account for situations where people, certain a remedy would work, see no effect, only to experience profound shifts with another remedy chosen later, often when they least expect it. This demonstrates that it is not about belief or intention; it is about the remedy being an energetic match. Homeopathy works beyond the placebo effect.

True Healing and Remedy Reactions

The next section explores:
- what healing looks like
- remedy reactions
- maintaining causes and blocks to cure.

What Does Healing Look Like?

Healing is not always an immediate disappearance of symptoms; instead, it can unfold according to certain principles, known as Hering's Law of Cure. Named after Dr. Constantine Hering, this law outlines the patterns of healing that may occur during homeopathic treatment as shown below.

These patterns recognise that some symptoms, like fever, serve a functional purpose in the body's healing process. Homeopathy supports and accelerates this natural healing by aligning with the body's innate processes rather than suppressing them.

Hering's Law of Cure

TOP TO BOTTOM
Symptoms may move from top to bottom, or from the centre to extremities. E.g. joint pains or rashes may move from shoulders to hips, then to legs.

FROM INSIDE TO OUTSIDE
Symptoms move from within to the outside. We must allow the body to cleanse and eliminate toxins without suppressing any kind of discharge.

 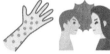

REVERSE ORDER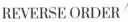
Old symptoms which have been suppressed or incompletely cured may return, and in the reverse order of their original appearance.

FROM MOST IMPORTANT TO LEAST IMPORTANT ORGANS
E.g. as depression/anxiety/panic attacks clears, the patient may develop symptoms on a physical level, such as, a rash or digestive disorders.

You feel better - pain and symptoms subside. You have more energy.

You may fall asleep - the body gets to work while you sleep and you wake up feeling better.

Elimination may occur - discharges such as mucus, diarrhoea, vomit, rashes, profuse urination or even words occur temporarily and you feel better afterwards.

Remedy Reactions

Herx and detox responses

In homeopathy, a detox response, also referred to as a healing crisis or Herxheimer ('herx') reaction, can occur when the body begins to heal and eliminate toxins. This temporary response often results in an intensification of symptoms, like fever, headache, muscle ache or fatigue. While uncomfortable, this reaction indicates that the remedy is effectively stimulating the body's detoxification process. It serves as a reminder that true healing involves the body's natural clearing of toxins, which may temporarily feel like a setback but ultimately leads to deeper recovery. The body needs to eliminate and unsuppress in order to heal. It is temporary and we feel better afterwards!

Return of old symptoms

This is similar to a herx reaction but subtly different. A 'return of old symptoms' is when old health issues return - these are issues which may have been previously suppressed or incompletely cured in the past. Typically, the body will prioritise more vital organs. For example, if a patient is being treated for asthma and previously had eczema (suppressed by steroids), the skin issues may return while the lungs heal. A return of old symptoms is a good thing and shows deep healing is taking place.

Proving remedies

If we repeatedly take a remedy when it is not needed, we risk proving the remedy—this means experiencing the symptoms that the remedy typically cures.

This is very rare in acute situations because the energy of the symptoms is strong, and the energy of a remedy that is not needed will generally bounce off. Although uncommon in chronic issues, provings can happen, which is one reason why self-treating chronic conditions is not recommended.

It is also why we must respect the homeopathic law of the minimum dose - less is more in homeopathy. Once healing has been stimulated, we don't need to keep taking the remedy unless healing stalls. However, provings are rare and typically cease once the remedy is stopped.

Remedy Reactions

Aggravations
True aggravations are uncommon. These are when symptoms worsen with no improvement. Normally, any worsening of symptoms is actually a herx reaction but it is important to look at this in the context of the total case. If there was an aggravation followed by improvement, then this is a good sign but teaches us that the potency may have been too strong.

Relapses
This is when the remedy has worked at some point and now the individual's vitality is going backwards. It may mean that the remedy needs repeating or the potency needs increasing. It is important to also look at whether there are interfering factors.

What if there is no change after taking the remedy?
If there has been absolutely NO change at all, then it could be due to one of the following possibilities:

- Were there any antidoting factors such as strong mint or coffee consumed after taking the remedy? Although some homeopaths say this is a possibility, I haven't ever seen this happen in practice.
- Could it simply have been the wrong remedy? It might be that some critical information wasn't obtained at the homeopathic consultation.
- Was it the right remedy but the potency was way off? This is unlikely as we would expect there to be some change, even if minor, with the 'right' remedy but 'wrong' potency.
- Could there be a block to cure? It might be that there are miasmatic influences or drug layers that need treating—see later chapters.
- Could there be maintaining causes? Is there a maintaining cause such as poor diet, toxic relationship or other external stressor such as a miserable job, which could be creating symptoms? Homeopathy can give the individual an energetic impetus to make changes in these regards, but ultimately it is up to their free will to make the final changes in their lives, and sometimes practicalities will make this difficult.

Maintaining Causes and Blocks to Cure

'Those diseases are improperly called chronic that are suffered by people who:

- continually expose themselves to avoidable malignities,
- habitually partake of harmful food or drink,
- abandon themselves to intemperances of all kinds, which undermine health,
- undergo prolonged deprivation of things that are necessary for life,
- live in unhealthy places,
- reside only in cellars, damp workplaces or other confined quarters,
- suffer lack of exercise or open air,
- deprive themselves of health by excessive mental or bodily exertions,
- live in constant vexation.

these kinds of ill-health that people bring upon themselves disappear spontaneously under an improved lifestyle, provided no chronic miasm lies in the body.'

Hahnemann - The Chronic Diseases: Their Peculiar Nature and Their Homoeopathic Cure

In homeopathy, the idea of 'maintaining causes' refers to ongoing factors in a person's environment, lifestyle or emotional landscape that continually challenge or weaken the vital force. Hahnemann was already aware of these in his time (as noted above), and he stated that some conditions are 'improperly called chronic' when they are, in fact, self-inflicted and maintained by the individual's choices and environment. He believed that these chronic conditions described above, could spontaneously improve if the underlying causes were removed, provided no deeper miasmatic influence was present.

This insight is profoundly empowering. It underscores that the power to heal often lies within the individual. While homeopaths offer guidance, we must not outsource our health to any healer, whether a homeopath or conventional doctor. True healing requires a commitment to actively engage in our own health journey.

Maintaining Causes and Blocks to Cure

Modern maintaining causes
Today, maintaining causes may encompass:
- Toxic relationships: Stress from unhealthy relationships can obstruct healing.
- Dissatisfying career or lack of purpose: Feelings of being unfulfilled or without direction can drain energy and block progress.
- Living environment: Poor air quality, dampness, mould and noise can continuously stress the body.
- Diet and water quality: Processed foods, toxins and inadequate hydration compromise well-being.
- Electromagnetic Fields (EMFs): New challenges like EMFs from electronic devices can disturb the body's energetic balance.
- Drug layers and genetic factors: Past medications or inherited predispositions (miasms) can block healing - explained in more detail in the next section.

When these are addressed, many symptoms of ill-health can disappear, sometimes without any remedy.

Recognising deeper blocks: Miasms and drug layers
While maintaining causes often require lifestyle changes, deeper blocks like miasms or drug layers may need targeted remedies. Miasms represent inherited or acquired tendencies toward certain health issues, while drug layers can stem from past medication use, creating energetic imprints that interfere with healing. Both of these will be explored further in this book in the next chapters.

The power of the individual
Embracing these concepts encourages us to take charge of our health by addressing our environment and lifestyle choices alongside selecting the right remedy. Homeopathy offers a guide, but we must make conscious choices—like what we eat and how we manage stress—to truly heal. This shift from passive to active participation in our well-being is not just empowering, it's crucial for achieving lasting health.

Miasms

The next section explores miasms, including:
- what are they?
- an exploration of energetic transfer.
- how miasms present in individuals?
- the emergence of a new miasm?
- a different perspective on childhood illnesses.

Miasms - Acquired Energy Patterns

When we talk about health and disease, both hereditary and environmental factors play a vital role. While traditional genetics focuses on how DNA determines our predisposition to certain conditions, it is becoming increasingly evident that inheritance involves much more than just genes. Epigenetics shows us that experiences, traumas and even diseases acquired in our lifetime can leave a profound imprint on future generations.

A study by Brian Dias and Kerry Ressler (2013) published in Nature Neuroscience demonstrated that trauma could be passed down epigenetically. Male mice conditioned to fear the smell of cherry blossoms by associating it with mild electric shocks had offspring that exhibited the same fear, despite never being exposed to the scent or the trauma. They concluded this inherited response was linked to changes in DNA methylation patterns on genes associated with scent receptors, showing that emotions can be encoded biologically and transmitted across generations. This research reminds us how our experiences shape us and our descendants.

Long before modern science recognised the concept of genetically-linked diseases, Hahnemann identified the phenomenon of inherited susceptibility, which he termed miasms. Originating from the Greek word for 'stain' or 'pollution,' miasms are seen as inherited or acquired dispositions that affect an individual's health across their lifetime. Hahnemann understood that the predisposition to certain health issues could be passed down through generations.

Our susceptibility is not only inherited; it is also profoundly shaped by what we encounter in our own lifetimes. Trauma, toxins and medications, to name just a few factors, can deeply influence our energetic field and thereby our predisposition to physical issues.

Reflect on the experiences of the last few years in relation to the 'Covid-19 Pandemic'. Almost no one can deny the emotional weight we've all felt—whether it was the fear of contagion, the fear of losing freedoms or the anger and frustration from feeling censored. These intense emotions don't just fade away; they linger and can lay down an energetic foundation that could manifest as 'symptoms' in the future—both in our own lives and in the lives of those who come after us. If we 31

Miasms - Acquired Energy Patterns

don't actively work to clear these energetic patterns, they remain, influencing our health and well-being.

When we carry the energy of miasms, they can create a tendency toward specific symptoms or types of illnesses. This is why sometimes we see even infants and babies, who have never been exposed to certain pathogens or traumas, presenting with chronic illnesses and disease. It is the inherited energetic blueprint, shaped by the miasms, that predisposes them to such conditions.

Homeopathy recognises five major chronic miasms, each carrying its own set of susceptibilities to specific illnesses, with considerable overlap between them. Hahnemann initially identified three primary miasms: Psora, Sycosis and Syphilis, and over time other homeopaths have expanded on Hahnemann's theories, introducing additional miasms like the Tubercular and the Cancer miasms.

The miasmatic remedies themselves are made in the same way as other homeopathic remedies but their original source material are the originating diseases. We call homeopathic remedies made from diseases 'nosodes'—remember though that homeopathic remedies do not contain any molecule of the original substance out of which they were made, they only contain the energetic imprint. Each miasm has its characteristic manifestations, which are explored on pages 134-145.

Let's explore in a little more detail how we acquire miasms. Miasms can either be inherited or acquired in one's own lifetime.

1) Inherited miasms
Inherited miasms are quite simply the energetic imprints of disease states that are passed down from one generation to the next. We are all born with varying degrees of all the miasmatic states (which might be active or dormant as explained on pages 36 and 37).

2) Miasms acquired during one's lifetime
Miasms are not only inherited but can also be acquired during our own lifetime. Our experiences, traumas, and even our relationships, leave deep imprints on our vital force, creating new miasmatic tendencies that may also be passed down to future generations.

Miasms - Acquired Energy Patterns

Miasms acquired in one's own lifetime may be 'infective' or 'non-infective' as described below:

- Infective miasms - An infective miasm can be acquired following an acute illness. For example, an individual might notice that they have 'never been well since' recovering from tuberculosis. In this case, the energetic imprint of the tuberculosis experience creates a chronic predisposition in that person where they are prone to say, respiratory issues and allergies. This energetic pattern is not confined to their lifetime but may also be passed on to the next generation, even when there is no discernible change in the parent's DNA. It is the vibrational memory of the disease that persists and is transferred.

- Non-infective miasms - Non-infective miasms may be acquired indirectly through what could be described as energetic transfer. Consider the case of a woman who starts experiencing recurrent cystitis after entering into a relationship with a new partner who previously had gonorrhoea (even though it was treated with antibiotics prior to them getting together). Over time, she develops fibroids, and her child with this partner is later affected by conditions such as glue ear and warts. There is no bacterial transmission here; what we are witnessing is the acquisition of the sycotic miasm – an energetic imprint transferred from one individual to another (Tabrett 2017).

The exact mechanism behind this energetic transfer may not yet be fully understood by contemporary science, but its effects are observable in clinical practice. This invites us to look beyond what is seen and measured, recognising the hidden influences that affect our health.

Understanding Energetic Transfer

Linking miasms and the Kaznacheev experiment: A deeper understanding of energetic transfer

These observations of miasm acquisition connect beautifully with the groundbreaking work of Russian biophysicist Vlail Kaznacheev, who in 1980 demonstrated that cells could communicate and influence each other at a distance without direct contact. His experiment, 'Distant Intercellular Electromagnetic Interaction,' revealed that when one culture of cells was exposed to harmful agents such as toxins, a second culture, kept separate but optically connected in quartz containers, began to show similar pathological changes—even though no direct physical contact occurred.

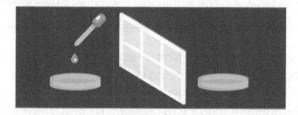

Kaznacheev's findings may suggest that cells can communicate via an electromagnetic field within the ultraviolet spectrum, enabling a 'biophotonic' exchange of information. This research may indicate that an energetic transfer can occur without any material or biochemical exchange. It mirrors the phenomenon we observe in homeopathy, where the imprint of a disease state, or miasm, can be passed on energetically, much like the woman acquiring the sycotic miasm from her partner.

Kaznacheev's work gives us a scientific lens through which we can explore the concept of miasmatic influence and the subtle energetic fields that connect all living beings. His findings support what we observe in practice—that diseases, symptoms and predispositions can be transmitted in ways that transcend the physical and biochemical. They may occur through a vibrational memory or energetic signature that penetrates deeply into the individual's energetic matrix, creating a predisposition to certain patterns of health or disease.

[1] I first heard of the Kaznacheev experiment during Alec Zeck's speech at the "What if My Body is Brilliant?" event, which I hosted in London in August 2024.

Understanding Energetic Transfer

Understanding these electromagnetic interactions deepens our appreciation of how health, disease and healing occur on levels far more subtle than we previously imagined. It highlights the importance of energetic hygiene, conscious relationships and awareness of the unseen impacts of our interactions with others.

Homeopathy has always recognised the profound interconnectedness of all living beings and the powerful implications of energetic exchanges that defy conventional biomedical paradigms.

Kaznacheev's work suggests that such transfers may not require the physical exchange of bacteria or viruses; instead, the disease's energetic essence—its vital force disturbance—is transmitted through subtle electromagnetic fields. It is a transfer of information, not in the classical Newtonian sense, but in a more quantum and vibrational framework, where the informational content of the miasm penetrates deeply into the individual's energetic matrix.

This aligns with homeopathic principles, where the remedy works not by direct biochemical intervention but by providing a resonant energetic signature that assists the body's vital force in restoring homeostasis and wellness.

How Do Miasms Show Up?

So, finally, how will miasms be clinically indicated in individuals?
There are three ways in which miasms may be clinically indicated in individuals as explained below.

1. Exposed miasm

This is when the totality of the patient's case matches the corresponding miasmatic remedy - i.e. on a mental, emotional and physical level. There is also evidence of the miasm in the patient's family medical history. The miasmatic remedy is prescribed in the same way as any other 'constitutional' remedy.

To illustrate, imagine an individual who has always been prone to skin issues, particularly eczema, which flare up during times of stress. Mentally and emotionally, she has a sense of lack, especially around money, and tends to worry excessively, which often exacerbates her skin condition. A detailed look into her family medical history reveals a pattern: her mother suffered from severe allergies and her grandfather had psoriasis.

In this case, the Psoric miasm is clearly exposed, as the symptoms align perfectly on a mental, emotional and physical level across generations. The homeopathic practitioner chooses Psorinum. This acts as a constitutional remedy, aiming to heal the individual's chronic conditions by addressing the deep-seated miasmatic influences.

2. Active miasm

This is when the miasm is actively producing a tendency to certain health issues and when well-indicated constitutional remedies fail to act. There is likely to be evidence of the miasm in the patient's family medical history.

For example, consider another scenario with an individual who has recurring respiratory issues and a history of tuberculosis in his family. Despite receiving well-indicated constitutional remedies like Phosphorus for his lung issues, his condition only shows temporary improvement, with symptoms quickly resurfacing. This suggests an active Tubercular miasm, where the underlying miasmatic influence is actively disrupting his health, leading to a continuous cycle of illness

36

How Do Miasms Show Up?

despite appropriate remedies. In this case, the practitioner might choose to give the miasmatic remedy Tuberculinum, which directly addresses the Tubercular miasm, aiming to break the cycle of recurring symptoms.

3. Dormant miasm
The is where the miasm is indicated in the patient's family history or previous illnesses, but there is no evidence the miasm is active.

To illustrate, let's look at a woman who sees a homeopath because she is concerned about her risk of developing arthritis since both her parents suffered from it in their later years. However, she currently shows no symptoms of arthritis or any related condition. Her overall health is good, and she has no other significant past illnesses that would indicate an active miasm.

In this situation, the Syphilitic miasm is considered dormant. The family history suggests a latent miasmatic influence but, with no active symptoms, most homeopaths, following traditional practice, would not treat her for this dormant miasm. The focus would instead be on maintaining her good health without delving into miasmatic treatment unless clear symptoms manifest.

The nosodes relating to miasms are under-represented in homeopathic repertories, making it essential for homeopaths to have an excellent knowledge of these deep-acting remedies. Miasmatic remedies should not be self-prescribed due to their powerful, far-reaching effects and the expertise needed to apply them appropriately.

The Emergence of a 'Strep' Miasm?
And a new childhood epidemic

Over time, the repeated suppression of Streptococcus with antibiotics may have given rise to a new miasm—one marked by chronic and lingering patterns of illness that defy conventional treatment. As society aggressively treated strep throat with antibiotics and, in extreme cases, tonsillectomies, we may have inadvertently pushed the energetic imprint of this acute illness deeper into the body's vital force, creating a hidden susceptibility.

We are now witnessing a surge in cases of PANDAS (Pediatric Autoimmune Neuropsychiatric Disorders Associated with Streptococcal Infections), with up to 1 in 200 children estimated to be affected. This was one of the most common complaints I encountered in my clinic. In PANDAS, children suddenly develop neuropsychiatric symptoms like OCD, separation anxiety, sensory issues, regression and/or tics, which mainstream medicine links to 'strep infections' (though it's important to note that the root cause often goes much deeper, as not all children with strep develop PANDAS). The concerning rise in PANDAS may point to an underlying miasmatic influence, where the suppressed energy of the strep bacteria triggers profound behavioural and mental health disturbances.

By recognising strep as a potential new miasm, we acknowledge that the body's response to this bacterial imprint has shifted from acute, manageable symptoms to deeper chronic patterns affecting the mind and emotions. To help clear the energetic imprint, homeopathy offers the remedy Streptococcinum (see page 144). Just as we use Psorinum to address the underlying susceptibility of the psoric miasm, Streptococcinum can be employed to help target the lingering energetic patterns associated with the suppression of strep symptoms.

It is important to note, however, that the treatment of children with PANDAS typically involves a multi-layered approach including essential constitutional treatment, homeopathic detox, organ support as well as addressing miasms. Homeopathy offers a way to work with the body's vital force to release the suppressed imprint and restore balance rather than continuing the cycle of suppression and manifestation.

Childhood Illnesses
What if nature provided us with a way to clear these miasms...?

Consider the possibility that childhood illnesses are not merely random occurrences but nature's way of helping us clear inherited miasmatic imprints. These energetic patterns predispose us to certain diseases, so illnesses like chickenpox, measles and mumps may help release these deep-seated tendencies within the body.

For example, chickenpox, often seen in childhood, aligns with the psoric miasm, which is linked to a susceptibility to skin conditions, allergies and sensitivities. Experiencing chickenpox may help expel impurities from the body and build resilience—this is supported by studies which have shown that natural chickenpox may reduce the risk of certain cancers later in life (Canniff et al., 2011; Silverberg et al., 2012).

Measles relates to the syphilitic miasm, which involves a destructive tendency within the body, such as tissue breakdown or severe chronic conditions. By undergoing measles, the body may be purging deeper taints, potentially offering a protective effect, as seen in the lower incidence of cervical cancer in those who have had natural measles (Ronne, 1985).

Mumps, characterised by glandular swelling, corresponds to the sycotic miasm, which is associated with growths, excesses and chronic inflammation. Research suggests that girls who have had mumps have a reduced risk of ovarian cancer (West, 1996), indicating that this illness may help clear sycotic tendencies from the body.

These childhood illnesses could represent natural opportunities for the body to address and clear inherited energetic imprints, fostering deeper health and resilience. Observations also show that children often make developmental leaps following recovery from such illnesses, highlighting their potential role in promoting growth and transformation.

By recognising these 'illnesses' as part of our energetic evolution, we see nature's wisdom in guiding our journey toward greater health and well-being.

Sarcodes

The next section explores sarcodes - remedies made from healthy tissues or secretions, intended to support and balance corresponding tissues or functions in the human body.

Sarcodes
When our organs need a helping hand...

Sarcodes are a unique and vital category of homeopathic remedies, derived from healthy tissues, glands and secretions of the body. Sarcodes work by gently reminding the body how to function optimally. They are like tuning forks, resonating with specific organs or systems, helping them return to their natural state.

What are sarcodes?
Sarcodes are potentised homeopathic remedies that originate from healthy animal tissues, organs or their secretions, such as hormones or enzymes to help stimulate the body's inherent healing mechanisms. O.A. Julian (1979), in his foundational work, Materia Medica of New Homeopathic Remedies, highlighted how sarcodes could support the body's functions without replacing them. The goal is not to mimic or substitute the action of the tissue but to energetically stimulate it to regain its natural role.

How sarcodes work
The primary purpose of a sarcode is to balance and restore function. For example, if a patient has a sluggish thyroid, a homeopath might use the sarcode Thyroidinum, derived from thyroid tissue, to remind the thyroid gland of its normal function. This approach can be especially useful when the body has 'forgotten' how to regulate itself due to chronic illness, stress or aging. By using sarcodes, we aim to activate the body's natural healing abilities, allowing it to reset and return to harmony.

Dosing and potency guidelines
When using sarcodes, potency and dosing depend on the nature of the imbalance and the individual's sensitivity. Lower potencies, such as 3x or 4c, are often used to gently nudge the tissue into action, while higher potencies, like 30c, are suited for a more systemic and dynamic effect. For chronic conditions, sarcodes may be administered weekly or biweekly, whereas acute situations may require more frequent dosing, even daily. Dosing must always be tailored to the individual's specific health issues and vitality.

Sarcodes

When our organs need a helping hand...

Applications of sarcodes

Sarcodes are often employed in cases where an organ or tissue is not performing optimally but is not yet entirely dysfunctional. Here are some scenarios where sarcodes may be indicated:

- Endocrine support: Remedies like Thyroidinum for thyroid balance or Adrenalinum for adrenal fatigue.
- Hormonal rebalancing: Sarcodes such as Testosterone or Folliculinum may be used to address hormonal imbalances, helping the body remember how to regulate hormone production naturally.
- Immune function: Thymuline is commonly used to strengthen the immune response, especially during times of stress or seasonal changes.

When to use sarcodes

- To restore function: When an organ or tissue requires a gentle reminder of its job, such as supporting adrenal health in burnout cases.
- As part of a detox: During detoxing, sarcodes can help create a clearer pathway for detoxification and recovery. After clearing toxins, sarcodes can help organs like the liver or kidneys regain their natural function.
- To complement constitutional treatment: When a patient's constitutional remedy is not acting fully, sarcodes can help clear the pathway for its action.

Practical considerations

When prescribing sarcodes, we always consider the individual's overall health, vitality and response to other treatments. Because they support on a more physical level, we may wish to start with low potencies, monitoring for any signs of aggravation or improvement. Remember, the goal is not to replace the function of the tissue but to support and heal it, allowing the body to find its own balance once more.

Nosodes

The next section explores nosodes - remedies made from diseased tissue or bodily secretions associated with a particular illness.

Nosodes

A nosode is a type of homeopathic remedy prepared from pathological specimens, such as diseased tissues, bodily secretions or microorganisms associated with a particular illness. The preparation undergoes the homeopathic process of serial dilution and succussion to remove any toxic effects while retaining the energetic imprint of the original substance.

Homeopaths may use nosodes in various contexts:

- **Constitutional remedies**: Nosodes can be used as regular constitutional remedies when the individual's overall spiritual, emotional and physical state match the energy pattern of the nosode. For example, Lyssinum (a remedy made from the saliva of a rabid dog) is characterised by extreme fear of water, heightened sensitivity to light and noise, impulsiveness and intense anxiety and would be used when the patient's symptoms are a match.
- **'Never been well since'**: Nosodes are also effective when there is a clear history of 'never been well since' a particular illness. For instance, Influenzinum may be considered for someone who has never fully recovered from 'flu' symptoms. Here, nosodes help release the lingering energetic imprint of that disease, allowing the body to return to its natural state of balance.
- **Homeoprophylaxis:** Moving beyond individual cases, nosodes play a key role in homeoprophylaxis—using highly diluted preparations to strengthen the body's defense against specific diseases, as explored in more detail over the next few pages.
- **Miasms** - nosodes are used to remove miasmatic influences, as discussed previously.

By recognising the potential of nosodes to address both existing health imbalances and strengthening the vital force, to prevent future illness, we see a powerful tool that aligns with homeopathy's core principle: treating the individual as a whole, working at the level of the vital force and viewing health and disease through an energetic lens. As we explore homeoprophylaxis further in the next pages, we delve deeper into how nosodes can shape a new paradigm for preventative healthcare.

Homeoprophylaxis

The next section explores how we can use homeopathy to prevent illness - what we call 'Homeoprophylaxis.'

Using Homeopathy to Prevent Illness

Homeoprophylaxis is a method that uses homeopathic remedies, to strengthen the body's vital force against specific diseases by introducing an energetic imprint of the pathogen usually in the form of a homeopathic nosode.

It is speculated that homeoprophylaxis works by stimulating the body's innate defense mechanisms, enhancing its ability to recognise and respond to potential 'threats' before they manifest physically.

This approach has been used for centuries and one of the most well known examples of this is the use of Influenzinum, a homeopathic nosode made from the secretions of individuals with 'influenza' symptoms, to help manage influenza outbreaks.

Homeopath Dr. John Clarke (1853-1931) observed that by introducing the energetic signature of influenza, the homeopathic remedy Influenzinum could help the body's vital force resist the onset of symptoms and maintain a state of health. Similarly, in other historical instances, homeoprophylaxis has been employed successfully during epidemics to mitigate disease spread and severity, with consistent reports of lowered incidence among those treated with these potentised remedies.

> Clarke recommended the use of Influenzinum 'as the routine remedy in epidemics. It may be given in the 12th or 30th potency... When "colds" appear in a family let all those who are unaffected take Arsenicum 3c thrice daily, and let the patients take Influenzinum 30c every hour or two. This generally prevents the spread of the trouble and clears up the colds, whether they are influenza or not.'
>
> Clarke acknowledges that this prophylactic protocol goes against individual prescribing and cautions 'Influenza has the property of developing old troubles and thus it takes an infinite variety of forms in different persons, so that Influenzinum need not be expected to cure all cases unaided, or indeed be appropriate in every case.'

Using Homeopathy to Prevent Illness

Modern evidence supports the effectiveness of homeoprophylaxis. In a landmark study conducted by Bracho et al. (2010), a large-scale homeopathic intervention using a Leptospirosis nosode showed significant success in controlling an epidemic in Cuba. Following severe flooding in three Cuban provinces in 2007, which dramatically increased the risk of Leptospirosis, a potentised homeopathic preparation made from dilutions of four circulating Leptospira strains was administered orally to 2.3 million people at high risk.

The results were compelling: in the regions where the nosode was given, there was an observed reduction in disease incidence that fell below the historical median, even independently of the usual correlation with rainfall. By contrast, non-intervention regions showed no such reduction in Leptospirosis cases. The study recorded a significant drop in incidence rates in the intervention areas, providing a stark comparison to historical data and suggesting that homeoprophylaxis may have contributed to reducing the expected number of cases by over 84%.

The implications of homeoprophylaxis are profound, particularly with respect to how we understand and approach disease prevention. Rather than focusing solely on external factors, this method invites a broader perspective, recognising that health and disease operate within an energetic continuum. By aligning with the body's biofield, homeoprophylaxis provides a gentle yet potent way to strengthen resilience against illness, emphasising balance and harmony as core tenets of wellbeing. The potential of this method to reshape public health approaches—by integrating energetic understanding with practical application—opens up exciting possibilities for more holistic, accessible and sustainable healthcare solutions.

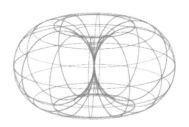

Homeoprophylaxis - Dosing

Dosing - prevention

The general standard practice of dosing nosodes to prevent symptoms during an epidemic or, for example, to prevent seasonal illness are:

- Take indicated remedy, e.g. Influenzinum for 'flu' or 'Pertussin' for whooping cough, in a 200c potency once a day for 1-3 days
- Repeat remedy every 2-4 weeks.

Is it necessary to always use a nosode to prevent disease?

No, it is not always necessary to use a nosode to prevent disease. It has been noted that in true epidemics, there is often a single remedy that best matches the energy of the disease. This dates back to Hahnemann's days when he used Belladonna to prevent Scarlet fever outbreaks.

> **Genus Epidemicus**
> 'a prescription based on Hahnemann's observation that during a true epidemic of acute disease, a majority of cases will respond to the same remedy, provided the remedy is similar to the characteristics of the epidemic.'
> Ian Watson
> A Guide to the Methodologies of Homeopathy

More recently during the Covid 19 Pandemic, the Indian Ministry of AYUSH (Ayurveda, Yoga & Naturopathy, Unani, Siddha, and Homeopathy) recommended Arsenicum 30c as the Genus Epidemicus —a homeopathic remedy believed to match the symptoms of the prevailing epidemic. Arsenicum was chosen based on its ability to address symptoms like anxiety, respiratory issues and gastrointestinal disturbances, which, according to allopathic medicine, were the most common Covid 19 symptoms.

Other common Genus Epidemicus remedies include Rhus Tox for chicken pox, Pulsatilla for measles, Drosera for whooping cough, Arsenicum for flu and Belladonna for Scarlet fever.

It is down to personal preference and experience as to whether a homeopath uses the nosode or, if there is one, the Genus Epidemicus remedy.

The Bowel Nosodes

The next section explores a specific class of nosodes called 'the bowel nosodes' - these are homeopathic remedies made out of gut bacteria - a very important group of remedies for the times we live in.

The Bowel Nosodes

I will be forever indebted to the bowel nosode Proteus, which, as I mentioned previously, triggered such an incredible and instant healing response in my daughter that I felt like I had witnessed a miracle. I was so awestruck with what I saw that I knew I had to learn more and so, not being one to do things by halves, I signed up to study homeopathy professionally.

As previously discussed, nosodes are homeopathic remedies made out of diseased tissue, pathogens or bodily secretions associated with a particular illness. Bowel nosodes are a specialised group of nosodes which are created from part of the bacterial flora in the human intestine.

> 'In spite of the name, the bowel nosodes are not similar agents to other nosodes, and do not act in the same way. Other nosodes act on a disease situation, either as part of treatment in the acute illness, or to address the energetic imprint of that illness, or to correct imbalances in the 'soil' of potential sufferers. In contrast, the bowel nosodes, with their source material being the result of a healing reaction in the body, act at the curative end of the 'dis-ease' spectrum and augment that curative action.'
>
> John Saxton - Bowel Nosodes in Homeopathic Practice

Bowel nosodes were discovered by Dr. Edward Bach (1886–1936), a renowned bacteriologist at University College Hospital, London. You could say Dr. Bach was ahead of his time. While modern science now recognises the importance of gut health and its connection to mental well-being, Dr. Bach had inklings of this as early as the 1920s. He noticed that high levels of certain bacteria in his patients' stool samples correlated with specific health issues. His curiosity led him to accept a position at the London Homeopathic Hospital, where he encountered homeopathic principles. Collaborating with Dr. John Paterson and Dr. Charles Wheeler, he began creating homeopathic preparations from intestinal bacteria, which became known as the bowel nosodes.

Dr. Bach's work was groundbreaking, suggesting that the balance of bacteria in the gut could influence overall health—a concept now widely accepted.

The Bowel Nosodes

Bowel nosodes are generally used when there is a deep-rooted imbalance affecting both body and mind. Homeopaths often turn to these remedies when symptoms persist despite other treatments, such as constitutional or miasmatic remedies. This wonderful group of remedies are amazing at treating a whole range of issues, including **bowel, digestive, lung, skin and immune system issues** as well as **toxicity** and **emotional disorders**.

They are valuable for patients experiencing mental tension, anxiety or feelings of being 'stuck,' often linked to a toxic or imbalanced gut environment.

By addressing the gut—the body's 'second brain'—bowel nosodes help realign the body's energetic field, promoting harmony and resilience across both physical and emotional health. This approach recognises that disturbances in the microbiome can mirror and perpetuate deeper emotional and physical states, making bowel nosodes a potent tool in restoring balance and health holistically.

There are 13 core bowel nosodes, each with their own specific picture as detailed on pages 178-197.

When are bowel nosodes prescribed?
- As a constitutional remedy in their own right, but note these remedies are hugely under-represented in the Repertories, so it is essential that the homeopath has an excellent knowledge so they can spot them in their patients.
- As an intercurrent remedy to address obstacles or blocks that prevent the patient's primary remedy from working effectively.
- To help produce a clearer symptom picture - for example, to help clear a drug layer (say where there has been a history of excessive antibiotics) or where it is difficult to differentiate between multiple constitutional remedies which may be suitable.
- When well-indicated remedies fail to act or to hold.

The bowel nosodes are generally only prescribed by professional homeopaths for chronic states of ill health, on the individual's specific symptoms and health history.

Homeopathic Detox

This final section explores 'homeopathic detox' - this is an absolutely essential method of homeopathy for the current toxic times that we live in.

Homeopathy Detox for our Toxic World

> 'All schools within homeopathy aim to cure by triggering the self healing mechanism of the body. People without any allopathic medications in their history respond beautifully to a totality prescription. Unfortunately most people have been treated with medications or have come in contact with chemicals and toxic substances. These days, in the majority of cases, classical homeopathic remedies alone do not suffice to permanently neutralise present day external influences'
>
> Ton Jansen - Fighting Fire With Fire

Homeopathic detox addresses the side effects of toxins, drugs or other harmful substances. Unlike conventional detoxification approaches that focus only on the physical removal, homeopathic detox works at a deeper level, engaging the body's innate healing ability to clear these imprints both physically AND energetically.

Even when a substance has left the physical body, its energetic imprint can remain, causing disturbances in the body's vital force. For example, a medication taken years ago may have been physically excreted, but its energetic impact can still create blockages or symptoms that hinder healing. For example, think about the woman who, despite having stopped the contraceptive pill years ago, still hasn't had her periods return to 'normal', even though the physical drug left her system years ago. Homeopathic remedies made from the original toxin shine a spotlight on the residual imprint, signalling to the vital force to recognise and clear it.

I imagine some of you reading this are thinking 'but can't a well chosen constitutional solve all our health issues?' Trust me, I thought that too. What a marvellous idea that one remedy could shift the entire landscape of our health. But in today's toxic world, where layers of pollutants, medications and environmental stressors accumulate, our vital force sometimes needs extra help. Homeopathic detox acknowledges these layers, targeting them directly to clear the path, allowing constitutional remedies to act more fully and effectively, aligning with our body's innate healing potential. My own personal experience was that while my eczema was 80% better with constitutional homeopathy, it only fully healed once I had detoxed steroids, the medication which I originally took to suppress the eczema symptoms many years earlier.

Homeopathy Detox for our Toxic World

Now for a quick couple of definitions, as this form of homeopathy may also be referred to as isopathy or tautopathy:
- **Isopathy** - is prescribing a remedy made from the supposed causative agents of a disease.
- **Tautopathy** - 'is really a variation of isopathy, the difference being that tautopathy refers specifically to the prescription of a potentised drug or toxin that a person has ingested at some time previously' (Watson 2004).

When to use homeopathic detox
- When a patient has 'never been well since' taking a specific drug or toxin.
- When well-indicated constitutional remedies do not produce the desired effects and there is a history of toxin exposure.
- To support drug withdrawal (always under the supervision of the prescribing healthcare provider).
- When the drug or toxin is the direct cause (aetiology) of the patient's complaints.

What would Hahnemann have thought of homeopathic detox?
Back in Hahnemann's day, the environmental and chemical toxins were minimal compared to what we face today. Our modern world is flooded with pollutants, pharmaceuticals and chemicals that burden our bodies in unprecedented ways. Homeopathic detox has become crucial in today's toxic environment, where toxins like endocrine disruptors, heavy metals and synthetic chemicals are omnipresent.

Having said that, Hahnemann often applied the principles of isopathy, such as using Mercurius for mercury poisonings. Another notable example involved his artist friend, who had been unwell for some time, with various remedies failing to help. The artist, regularly using sepia (cuttlefish ink) in his work, had developed a habit of licking the end of his paintbrush, ingesting small amounts of the ink. Hahnemann recognised that his symptoms mirrored those produced by Sepia, which he had previously studied in homeopathic provings. The previous remedies had failed because they didn't address the condition caused by Sepia exposure. In a classic isopathic approach, Hahnemann potentised Sepia into a homeopathic remedy. After administering it, his

Homeopathy Detox for our Toxic World

friend's condition improved, demonstrating the effectiveness of treating symptoms with the very substance that caused them.

Hahnemann was a visionary and progressive thinker who continuously refined his ideas throughout his lifetime. He wrote six editions of the Organon of Medicine, each reflecting his evolving understanding of homeopathy. Given his willingness to adapt and embrace new insights, I think it is likely that Hahnemann would have supported modern approaches like homeopathic detox, recognising the need to address the unique challenges of today's toxic environment while staying true to homeopathy's core principles.

My approach to homeopathic detox
Utilising and inspired by Ton Jansen's 'Human Chemistry' method, outlined in his pioneering books 'Fighting Fire with Fire' and 'Human Chemistry Integrated Therapy'—I find it effective to use a layered approach to homeopathic detox. This process involves clearing one or multiple layers of toxicity at a time, in line with Jansen's Hierarchy, taking into account the individual's overall case, current state of health, and medical history.

Ton Jansen's Hierarchy, as described in more detail in his books, prioritises clearing mRNA products and toxins that impact the hormonal system, such as steroids and hormonal contraceptives, followed by other layers of toxins like vaccinations, antibiotics, chemicals and narcotics, while supporting the body's detox pathways and treating the individual's constitution throughout the process.

As well as the relevant isopathic detoxification remedies given over several months, generally I would also prescribe a constitutional remedy as well as remedies to support the detoxification process and organs, such as sarcodes, or a general supportive remedy like Golden Spiral. It is very important that we always respect the foundational homeopathic principles and treat the individual—the above is guidance not law.

Homeopathy Detox for our Toxic World

It is strongly recommended to ALWAYS work with an experienced homeopath for homeopathic detox. I have suffered personally with aggravations when detoxes were attempted in the 'wrong' order outside of Jansen's Hierarchy. Homeopathic detox can have strong reactions and aggravations when attempted without professional input or when detox pathways are not properly opened.

A Note on Contagion

Terrain theory posits that the body's internal environment, or 'terrain', determines its susceptibility to disease, rather than the germs themselves. When the body's terrain is balanced and healthy, pathogens cannot take hold. James Tyler Kent echoed this view when he stated in the quote above that the tuberculosis bacteria are 'the results of the disease' rather than its cause. He believed that microbes are merely expressions of an internal imbalance, suggesting that true healing comes from strengthening the body's vital force, not just eliminating germs.

Homeopathic detox complements the principles of terrain theory. By using homeopathic remedies derived from toxins or pathogens, like bacteria or mould, we work to clear their energetic imprints, bringing the body's terrain back into balance.

This process recognises that true healing happens by strengthening the body's own vitality, clearing obstacles and re-establishing equilibrium. This approach is especially relevant when dealing with 'never been well since' cases, where detoxification opens the door for constitutional remedies to take effect.

Homeopathic remedies made out of pathogens such as, for example, bacteria or mould, can help remove the 'energetic imprint' of the same substance. But once this has been 'cleared', we still always need to question why the individual's terrain got out of homeostasis in the first place - what made them susceptible? And this is where constitutional homeopathy comes into its own.

A Note on Contagion

Some of you familiar with terrain theory might be curious about homeopathic remedies made from 'viruses,' like Influenzinum, often used for those who have 'never been well since' flu symptoms. But how does this fit with the debate over whether viruses have truly been isolated? How can a remedy come from a 'flu virus' that may not exist as we've been taught?

Let's clarify: the homeopathic remedy for 'flu' isn't derived from a virus itself. It's made from the sputum of someone with 'flu-like symptoms,' then diluted and succussed to create a potentised nosode. Through the principle of 'like cures like,' it can trigger healing when given to someone experiencing similar symptoms. Many homeopathic remedies derived from diseases are prepared in this way.

If you're ready to rethink the mainstream narrative about 'catching' germs, check out the eye-opening books 'Can You Catch a Cold?' by Daniel Roytas and 'What Really Makes You Ill' by Dawn Lester and David Parker. These excellent and very well-referenced books challenge the conventional understanding of illness.

After all, we don't believe yawns are caused by a virus or bacteria, yet they are 'contagious,' much like women's menstrual cycles syncing up. Could this same energetic phenomenon apply to 'transmissible' illnesses? Food for thought.

Remedies for the 21st Century & Beyond

The 35 remedies in this next section, alongside the 77 from my first book, are among the most essential remedies for the times we face today. Never before have we encountered such widespread exposure to toxins, with mental health challenges at an all-time high, and a surge in behavioural issues and developmental conditions in children. The remedies presented here are particularly attuned to these modern issues, yet their scope extends far beyond.

I've maintained the familiar format you've grown to love from my first book, while also expanding on the mental and emotional aspects of each remedy. Additionally, where relevant, I have introduced new sections on dreams—an important element in remedy selection—and food affinities. All 'related remedies' that are noted at the end of each remedy are either included in this or my first book.

Remedies covered include:
- Alumina
- Amniotic Fluid
- Aurum
- Ayahuasca
- Baryta Carb
- Bismuth
- Borax
- Bufo
- Cannabis
- Coffea
- Cygnus cygnus
- Emerald
- Fluor Ac
- Golden Spiral
- Hura
- Hyoscymus
- Lac Caninum
- Lac Maternum
- Oscillococcinum
- Peregrine falcon
- Placenta
- Platina
- Plutonium
- Rad Brom
- Spectrum
- Saccharum
- Sanguinaria
- Scorpion
- Shungite
- Sol
- Tarentula
- Umbilical Cord
- Veratrum
- Vernix
- X-Ray

Alumina
Dementia

 FULL NAME: Aluminum Oxydata
Other names: Aluminium Oxide
Made from aluminium metal.

MENTAL SYMPTOMS:

- Weak memory
- Dementia, senility, memory loss
- Forgets things
- Loses one's way
- Timid
- Slow or vague responses
- Changeable moods
- Contrary
- Cannot be hurried
- Time passes slowly
- Obstinate
- Grumbles
- Depressed
- Feels guilty - as if has committed a crime
- Things seem unreal
- Fears falling forwards
- Brain weakness
- Fear of knives

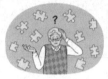

dementia   weak memory

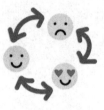 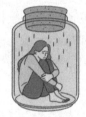

changeable   depressed
moods

EVENT THAT CAUSED SYMPTOMS:

- Aluminium toxicity
- Processed baby food
- Anger
- Disappointment

Alumina is derived from aluminium oxide and is often used to address symptoms associated with aluminium toxicity, such as mental confusion, sluggishness and a sensation of heaviness or paralysis, reflecting the remedy's link to aluminium's effects on the nervous system.

Alumina
Dementia

KEYNOTES & PHYSICAL SYMPTOMS:

- Aluminium poisoning
- Brain weakness and memory loss
- Dryness of mucus membranes
- Extreme constipation - feels compelled to use fingers to help evacuate
- Constipation in babies from artificial baby foods
- Colic especially when caused by heavy metals
- Vertigo upon waking
- Limbs feel heavy
- Progressive paralysis of limbs
- Feels like hot pokers were thrust through lower spine
- Dry, hacking morning cough
- Chronic head catarrh
- Needs to strain when doing stool to be able to urinate
- Brittle nails, old, dry, wrinkled skin
- Skin itches at night in bed
- Chronic blepharitis
- Scanty menses followed by exhaustion

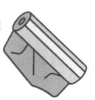

aluminium poisoning

memory loss

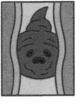

extreme constipation

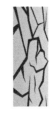

dry mucus membranes

warmth

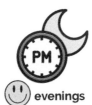

evenings

Hindered by:
Warmth of room or bed
Artificial food
Potatoes
Mornings
Speaking

Helped by:
Evenings
Damp weather
Cold
Washing
Open air

FOOD:

- No appetite - food has no taste
- Potatoes aggravate
- Desires starchy food

potatoes aggravate

no appetite

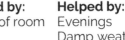

RELATED REMEDIES
Bryonia, Causticum, Opium, Sepia

Amniotic Fluid
Surrendering

 Other names: Amnii liquor
Made from amniotic fluid. This remedy is technically a sarcode but has been included in this section due to its wide scope of action.

MENTAL SYMPTOMS:
- This remedy enables us to surrender to the unknown
- Separation anxiety
- Fear of the new or uncertainty
- Anxious
- Feels unsupported or abandoned
- Dreamy or flakey
- Deep grief - as if drowning in grief
- Heightened senses
- Yearning for safety, security or a 'womb-like' environment
- May be ruthlessly independent
- Mental confusion or a sense of being lost
- Fear of dark water or drowning
- Feels intoxicated

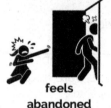

feels abandoned

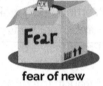

fear of new

grief

separation anxiety

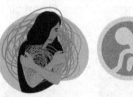

EVENT THAT CAUSED SYMPTOMS:
- Grief
- Abortion
- Miscarriage

This is a brilliant remedy to support individuals with anxiety. It can help the person to surrender and let go - putting faith and connection back to source and the higher self.

Amniotic Fluid
Surrendering

KEYNOTES & PHYSICAL SYMPTOMS:

- Low levels of amniotic fluid in pregnancy
- Babies who swallow meconium
- Death of twin in-utero (grief is in the waters)
- Colic and reflux in babies
- Breech babies
- Pneumonia where drowning in mucus
- Dry skin
- Insomnia
- Urinary issues including frequent urination
- Itchy eyes
- Hormonal issues
- One-sided headaches
- Palpitations

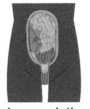

low amniotic fluid

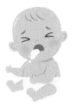

reflux

babies who swallow meconium

urinary issues

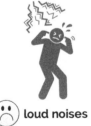

loud noises   warmth

Hindered by:
Bright lights
Loud noises
Sudden movements

Helped by:
Warmth
Enclosed spaces

FOOD:

- Cravings for soft food like porridge
- Desires milk

craves porridge

craves milk

RELATED REMEDIES
Natrum Mur, Placenta, Lac Humanum, Pulsatilla

Aurum
Dark night of the soul

FULL NAME: Aurum Metallicum
Other names: Gold
Made from the metal, gold.

MENTAL SYMPTOMS:
- Deep depression, despair or suicidal thoughts, especially when the person feels they have failed or are not living up to expectations
- Disgust of life
- High achievers and perfectionists who fear failure
- Intense feelings of responsibility - overwhelmed by duties and obligations
- Desires solitude
- Desire for meditation
- Self critical
- Feels worthless
- Tendency to be hard on oneself, with self-reproach, self-criticism or feelings of worthlessness
- Hopelessness
- Sensitive to contradiction - results in explosive anger
- Loves music

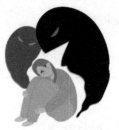

depressed and suicidal

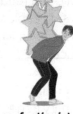

perfectionists

dutiful

loves music

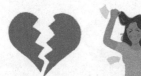

EVENT THAT CAUSED SYMPTOMS:
- Grief or disappointment in love
- Business failure
- Fright or anger
- LSD or MDMA abuse

Both Aurum and Tarentula have a deep connection to music: Aurum finds solace and healing in the soothing harmonies that calm their heavy hearts, while Tarentula craves the lively, rhythmic beats that fuel their restless energy and wild, unpredictable spirit.

Aurum
Dark night of the soul

KEYNOTES & PHYSICAL SYMPTOMS:

- Boring pains and burning stitches
- Heart issues - sensation as if heart stopped beating or palpitations
- Severe sinusitis
- Suffocative attacks
- High blood pressure
- Rush of blood to the head
- Ulcers which attack the bones
- Bone pains at night
- Infertility
- Chronic insomnia
- Moans in sleep
- Photophobia
- Oversensitive to pain
- Violent pain in head which is worse during the night
- Atrophy of testicles in boys
- Double vision or upper half of objects not visible

boring pains

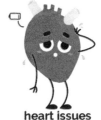
heart issues

high blood pressure

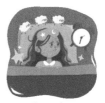
chronic insomnia

  night

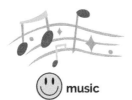 **music**

Hindered by:
Sunset to sunrise
Cloudy weather
Winter
Mental exertion

Helped by:
Open air
Cold bathing
Music
Walking
Evening

FOOD:

- Aversion to meat
- Loathing of food
- Desires alcohol, wine, milk, coffee

desires wine

loathes food

> **RELATED REMEDIES**
> Ignatia, Merc, Staphisagria, Sulphur, Syphilinum, Natrum Mur

Ayahuasca
Spiritual liberation

Made from the medicinal drug Ayahuasca, a hallucinogenic beverage, traditionally used by Indigenous cultures and folk healers in the Amazon and Orinoco basins for spiritual ceremonies.

MENTAL SYMPTOMS:

- Feeling of darkness
- Feels trapped in patterns or karmic ties
- Feeling spiritually 'stuck' or entangled in toxic relationships
- Extreme mood swings from rage to peace
- Heightened emotional sensitivity
- Disconnection from spiritual path - feels lost
- Vivid, compelling dreams that may reveal or resolve past traumas
- Sense of abandonment; longing for ancestral or personal reconnection
- Deep grief
- Fear of illness or cancer
- Hallucinations
- Self-hatred

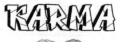

karmic ties

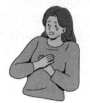

spiritually stuck

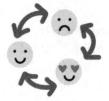

mood swings

fear of cancer

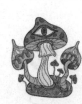

EVENT THAT CAUSED SYMPTOMS:

- Grief
- Long term use of hallucinogenic drugs

The Ayahuasca remedy was proved by the Guild of Homeopaths as part of their meditative proving series between 1992 and 1997.

Ayahuasca
Spiritual liberation

KEYNOTES & PHYSICAL SYMPTOMS:

- Deep fatigue, unrelieved by rest
- Heaviness or numbness in limbs
- Nausea, vomiting or diarrhoea worsened by stimulants
- Memory loss
- Respiratory problems, like constricted breathing or suffocation
- Neurological symptoms: tremors, tingling, 'flowing out' sensations
- Parkinson's or dementia
- Heightened sensory sensitivity
- Muscular weakness and soreness

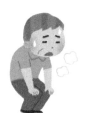
fatigue

heaviness in limbs

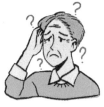
memory loss

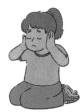
heightened senses

 night

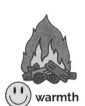
 warmth

Hindered by:
Night
Darkness
Isolation

Helped by:
Warmth

FOOD:

- Craves sweets and stimulants which aggravate

craves sweets and stimulants

> **RELATED REMEDIES**
> Arsenicum, Emerald, Golden Spiral, Spectrum

Baryta Carb
Developmental delays

 FULL NAME: Baryta Carbonica
Other names: Barium Carbonate Made from Barium Carbonate, a chemical compound consisting of barium, a heavy metal, combined with carbon and oxygen.

MENTAL SYMPTOMS:

- Slow mental grasp
- Developmental delays
- Childish
- Very shy and timid
- Bashful and very easily embarrassed
- Afraid of strangers
- Silly
- Poor concentration and weak memory
- Confusion
- Weak memory
- Senility and dementia
- Homesickness
- Lacking in confidence
- Fear of being laughed at
- Fear of change
- Poor at decision making
- Loss of mental functions after a stroke
- Anxiety especially about the future
- Conscientious
- Lacking independence
- Oversensitive
- Bites nails

timid

slow mental grasp

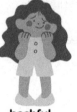

bashful

developmental delays

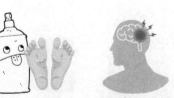

EVENT THAT CAUSED SYMPTOMS:
- Suppressed foot sweat
- Stroke

A remedy that is great for both children and in old age. It is one of the number 1 remedies for slow mental grasp.

Baryta Carb
Developmental delays

KEYNOTES & PHYSICAL SYMPTOMS:

- Glandular swellings
- Overweight individuals
- Children with large abdomen
- Slow growth
- Acts on the heart and vessels
- Gets cold easily
- Prostate swellings
- Prone to colds
- Offensive foot sweat
- Lipomas and fatty tumours
- Coughs after getting feet wet
- Crackling noise in ears
- Runny nose with swelling of nose and upper lip
- Tendency to tonsillitis
- Quinsy
- Aneurysm
- Weak digestion after eating
- Strong sense of smell

swollen glands

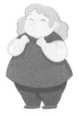
overweight

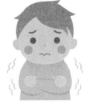
feels the cold

slow growth

mental exertion

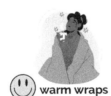
warm wraps

Hindered by:
Mental exertion
Emotions
Suppressed foot sweat
Cold

Helped by:
Open air
Warm wraps

FOOD:

- Loss of appetite
- Aversion to plums
- Better from cold food

loss of appetite

aversion to plums

RELATED REMEDIES
Ant Tart, Apis, Belladonna, Bufo, Calc Carb, Merc, Psorinum, Silica

Bismuth
'The Velcro Child'

 FULL NAME: Bismuthum Subnitricum
Other names: Magistrate of Bismuth
Made from a chemical compound of bismuth, a heavy metal, combined with nitric acid and water.

MENTAL SYMPTOMS:
- Known as 'the velcro kid' remedy (Chappell)
- Children cling to their mother's hand
- Fear of being alone - will follow parents everywhere
- Fear of death
- Depression, even suicidal
- Loss of power
- Irritable in daytime and better in the evening
- Extreme restlessness
- Anguish
- Unable to leave home
- Despair of recovery
- Unable to forgive
- Unstable and confused mind
- Often indicated where a friend or loved one has committed suicide - may have a sense of guilt around not being able to have helped

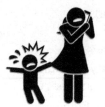

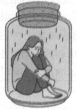

clingy   **depressed**

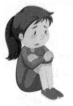

fear of being alone   **unable to leave home**

EVENT THAT CAUSED SYMPTOMS:
- Suicide of a loved one
- Loss of power

Very similar to Phosphorus and Arsenicum which sit in the same column as Bismuth in the Periodic Table.

Bismuth
'The Velcro Child'

KEYNOTES & PHYSICAL SYMPTOMS:

- Severe stomach pains
- Pain so great it causes writhing
- Burning, pinching or cramping pains
- Periodicity of symptoms
- Gastritis and stomach ulcers
- Headaches which appear mostly in winter
- Headaches alternating with stomach aches
- Vomiting large quantities of food
- Desires water which will then be vomited once it hits the stomach (like Phosphorus)
- Summer diarrhoea and watery stools
- Pale face with blue rings around eyes
- Flushes of heat especially over face and chest
- Low or lacking fever
- Infertility due to ovary issues
- Number 1 for cholera

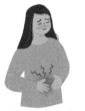 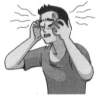

stomach pains   **headaches**

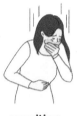 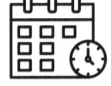

vomiting   **periodicity**

 being alone   **cold applications**

Hindered by:
Motion
Eating
Being alone
Summer
Winter

Helped by:
Cold applications
Cold drinks
Bending backwards

FOOD:

- Intolerable thirst
- Strong thirst for cold drinks which are vomited

extreme thirst   **cold drinks**

> **RELATED REMEDIES**
> Phosphorus, Arsenicum, Nux Vomica

Borax
Hypersensitivity

> **FULL NAME: Borax Veneta**
> **Other names: Sodium Biborate, Natrum Biboracicum**
> Made from sodium borate, a naturally occurring mineral.

MENTAL SYMPTOMS:

- Anxiety
- Very nervous and fearful
- Easily startled
- 'Dread of downward motion' - infant screams when laid down
- Fear of thunder and falling
- Hypersensitivity
- Sensitive to sudden noises even if at a distance
- Irritable
- Ill-humour
- Tendency to swear and curse
- Babies and children may shriek in sleep without any known reason
- Alternatively weeps and laughs
- Sleepiness
- Confusion - feels better after bowel movement
- Changes from one business or idea to another

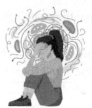 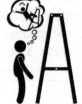

anxiety   fear of falling

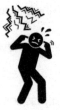 

sensitive to   easily
noises   startled

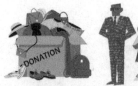 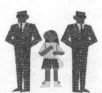

EVENT THAT CAUSED SYMPTOMS:

- Feeling used, exploited or trashed

'When Borax becomes important in a homeopathic treatment, a severe fungal infection is always present. The fungus and its host live together either in their mutual benefit or mutual dependency.'
Antonie Peppler - The Psychological Significance of Homeopathic Remedies

Borax
Hypersensitivity

KEYNOTES & PHYSICAL SYMPTOMS:

- One of the top remedies for oral thrush
- Extreme sensitivity
- General aggravation from descending
- Mouth ulcers which feel hot
- Herpetic eruptions
- Dry skin and psoriasis
- Galactorrhea (breast milk production unrelated to pregnancy or lactation)
- Infected or cracked nipples during nursing
- Headaches especially around 10am
- Shrieking before urinating
- Anxiety before stool
- Menses which are too frequent and yet profuse
- Leucorrhoea
- Sea and air sickness
- Useful in epilepsy
- Loose, offensive and pale stools

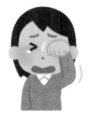 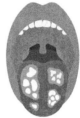

sensitivity　　**oral thrush**

mouth ulcers　　**leucorrhoea**

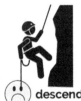

descending　**11pm**

Hindered by:
Descending
Before passing stool
10am

Helped by:
11pm
Cold weather
Pressure
After passing stool

FOOD:

- Loss of taste
- Desires sour food and acidic drinks
- Thirsty in the morning

loss of taste　**desires sour food**

RELATED REMEDIES
Natrum Mur, Merc, Apis

73

Bufo
Speech issues

FULL NAME: Bufo Rana
Other names: Toad poisoning Made from the poison expressed from the cutaneous glands on the back of the Bufo toad.

MENTAL SYMPTOMS:

- Buffoon like behaviour
- Delayed development including speech
- Anger if misunderstood
- Anxiety especially about health
- Fear of animals, strangers and mirrors
- Bites nails
- Nervous tics such as handwringing
- Babbling
- Loves music
- Loss of memory
- Mind remains childish even in older age
- Easily laughs or cries
- Bites or howls
- Desires solitude
- Deceitfulness

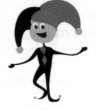

buffoon

anger when misunderstood

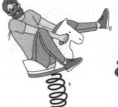

childish

developmental delays

EVENT THAT CAUSED SYMPTOMS:

- Shock
- Humiliation

The essence of Bufo can be seen in those whose intense inner turmoil manifests physically, from convulsions to spasmodic laughter, often without clear reason.

Bufo
Speech issues

KEYNOTES & PHYSICAL SYMPTOMS:

- Helps stimulate speech centres to help those with poor speech
- Slow development
- Poor muscle tone with floppiness
- Convulsions and spasms including epilepsy
- Oral issues - such as blowing raspberries or lapping tongue out (like the toad it is made from!)
- Stimming
- Colicky pains
- Tumours in breast with bloody discharges
- Headache with epilepsy
- Red streaks under the skin
- Infected carbuncles
- Impotence
- Excessive masturbation

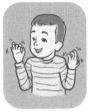

stimming

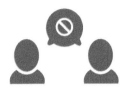

speech delays

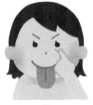

oral issues

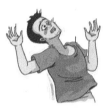

convulsions

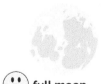

full moon

cold bathing

Hindered by:
Warm room
Sexual excitement
Full moon
On waking

Helped by:
Cold bathing
Bleeding
Putting feet in hot water

FOOD:

- Desires sweet drinks
- Loves brandy and getting drunk

desires sweet drinks

loves brandy

RELATED REMEDIES
Baryta Carb, Tarentula

Cannabis
Suppressed intuition

FULL NAME: Cannabis Indica
Made from from the Cannabis Indica plant, which typically has higher levels of THC than Cannabis Sativa, a different homeopathic remedy.

MENTAL SYMPTOMS:
- Suppressed intuition
- Suppresses own feelings in favour of others
- Distorted sense of space and time - time seems too long
- Disorientated
- Forgetful
- Sudden loss of memory
- Uncontrollable laughter
- Feels high
- Spaciness and out of body sensation
- Clairvoyance
- Chronic insomnia
- Paranoia
- Panic attacks
- Agitated, nervous and anxious
- Extremely chatty
- Fear of insanity
- Hallucinations

suppressed intuition   **distorted sense of time & space**

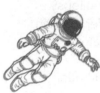

spaciness   **uncontrollable laughter**

EVENT THAT CAUSED SYMPTOMS:
- Cannabis use
- Parents who frequently used cannabis prior to conception

Cannabis Indica is predominantly used in homeopathy for addressing complex psychological and emotional conditions, whereas the remedy Cannabis Sativa is mainly used for physical ailments like urinary problems and mild mental disturbance

Cannabis
Suppressed intuition

KEYNOTES & PHYSICAL SYMPTOMS:

- Great desire to lie down in the daytime
- Easily exhausted
- Soothes nervous disorders like epilepsy, dementia and irritable reflexes
- Weak memory
- Nausea
- Unquenchable thirst
- Backache especially across shoulders and spine - must stoop
- Urinary disorders - urine dribbles and burns
- Profuse menses
- Feels as if top of head opens and closes
- Involuntary shaking of head
- Paralysis of lower limbs or limbs feel light
- Increased sexual desire
- Grinds teeth

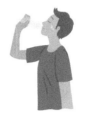
unquenchable thirst

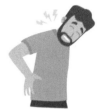
backache

urinary issues

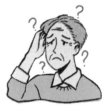
weak memory

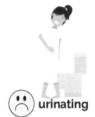

urinating

cold water

Hindered by:
Urinating
Darkness
Coffee
Night

Helped by:
Fresh air
Cold water
Rest

FOOD:

- Ravenous appetite
- Craves sweets
- Thirsty for cold drinks

ravenous

craves sweets

RELATED REMEDIES
Nitric Acid, Thuja, Sulphur, Phosphorus

Coffea
Overexcitability

FULL NAME: Coffea Cruda
Other names: Unroasted coffee
Made from the raw berries of coffee.

MENTAL SYMPTOMS:
- Overexcitability
- Hyperactivity of mind and body
- Restlessness
- Severe insomnia
- Full of ideas - quick to act on them
- Nervous agitation
- Hysteria
- Emotional reactivity - cries and laughs easily
- Intolerance of pain
- Fear of death from pains
- Fright from sudden but pleasant surprise
- Mind won't switch off in the evening
- Capricious
- Fainting from strong emotions
- Ecstatic states

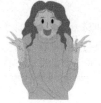
overexcitable

restless

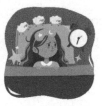

insomnia

emotional reactivity

EVENT THAT CAUSED SYMPTOMS:
- Fear
- Sudden pleasant surprises
- Disappointed love

Homeopathy uses two remedies from coffee: Coffea Cruda (raw coffee) for insomnia, overexcitement and sensitivity due to its stimulating effects, and Coffea Tosta (roasted coffee) for digestive issues and fatigue, highlighting different uses based on preparation.

Coffea
Overexcitability

KEYNOTES & PHYSICAL SYMPTOMS:

- Heightened sensitivity to touch, noise, odours
- Insomnia
- Sleeplessness due to a flow of ideas
- Stomach pains with despair
- Pressure in stomach
- Toothache helped by icy water in mouth
- Unendurable colic
- Sensitive hearing
- As if a nail driven into head
- Coffee headaches
- Pain that drives one to despair
- Palpitations
- Acute sensitive smell
- Hypersensitive vulva and vagina

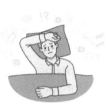
insomnia

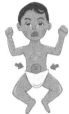
colic

toothaches

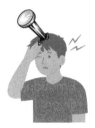
headache as if nail in head

 excitement

 cold drinks

Hindered by:
Excitement
Strong odours
Noise
Touch
Cold, wind

Helped by:
Warmth
Cold drinks
Lying down

FOOD:

- Aggravated by red wine, coffee
- Aversion to coffee

wine aggravates

averse to coffee

> **RELATED REMEDIES**
> Aconite, Ignatia, Pulsatilla, Natrum Mur, China, Ipecac

79

Cygnus Cygnus
Long-standing grief

Other name: Whooper swan
Prepared from a feather of the Whooper swan.

MENTAL SYMPTOMS:
- Long-standing crippling grief
- Feeling like an orphaned child, experiencing extreme loneliness
- Unable to connect and communicate
- Deep depression
- Irritability, anger, hatred and impatience
- Emotional outbursts
- Overwhelmed
- Fear of new things and open spaces
- Anxiety and paranoia about children's safety, financial security, future and health
- Difficulty with numbers and words, feeling like time moves slowly
- Sensitivity to artificial smells, chemicals, pollution and odours

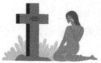

grief   **loneliness**

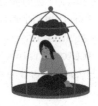

unable to **deep**
communicate **depression**

EVENT THAT CAUSED SYMPTOMS:
- Sexual abuse
- Being unwanted by their mother

DREAMS:
- Water and sea
- Pregnancy or childbirth
- Grief and isolation

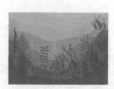

Cygnus Cygnus
Long-standing grief

KEYNOTES & PHYSICAL SYMPTOMS:

- Chest or throat issues
- Difficulty breathing or feeling of constriction
- Congested throat and may have much mucus
- Chest feels hollow
- Empty feeling in stomach
- Watery stools
- Sighing
- Heart feels constricted
- Nose often feels clogged
- Alternating low and high energy
- Symptoms may appear on alternating sides
- Poor circulation may have icy cold feet
- Short menstrual cycle
- Various types of rashes, blisters, red spots, warts or migratory itching

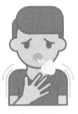
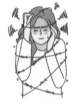

breathing issues **feeling of constriction**

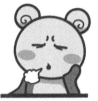

throat issues **sighing**

 2-5am **white**

Hindered by:
Afternoon
Evening
2-5am

Helped by:
Colour white

FOOD:

- Desires dark chocolate, stimulants, cola, coffee, spicy food, cigarettes
- Thirsty for water

desires chocolate and cola

RELATED REMEDIES
Natrum Mur, Ignatia, Staphisagria

81

Emerald
Helping one to let go

FULL NAME: Emerald
Prepared from the emerald gemstone.

MENTAL SYMPTOMS:
- Feels insecure and inadequate
- Gives one the strength to face suppressed emotional issues
- Calming effect on the mind
- Helps to let go of 'inhibiting emotions that are to do with parent-induced trauma' (Griffith)
- Grounding remedy - especially where the person is 'not in the body' (Griffith)
- Exhausted
- Mood swings
- Addictive personalities
- Bitterness from the past
- Unable to forgive
- Indecisive
- Desires sleep so that problems will disappear
- Can be confused with Natrum Mur as both are big grief remedies but Emerald is more willing to confront their grief

insecure

helps ground

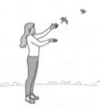

helps to let go

parent-induced trauma

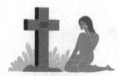

EVENT THAT CAUSED SYMPTOMS:
- Grief
- Abuse from parents
- Years of caregiving

Emerald is one of the 'new' remedies which was first proved by the Guild of Homeopaths in 1996.

Emerald
Helping one to let go

KEYNOTES & PHYSICAL SYMPTOMS:

- First remedy when any body part is to be extracted (e.g. teeth, warts, polyps, appendix etc) - 'helps the body to let go...without storing the memory of the trauma to the surrounding tissue' (Griffith)
- Reduces pain and surgical complications
- Major heart remedy
- Calms the nervous system
- Chronic fatigue
- PTSD
- Grief from sustained traumas
- Uterine problems after grief or trauma
- Feeling of not being in the body
- Debilitating nervous system disorders such after strokes
- Anti-radiation remedy
- Improves circulation and cleanses lymph

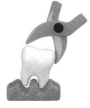 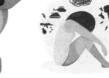

extractions   **PTSD**

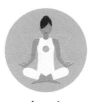 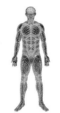

heart issues   **nervous system issues**

 night   **day**

Hindered by:
Night
Left side

Helped by:
Daytime

FOOD:

- Poor assimilation of food
- Desires limes and bitter fruit

 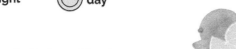

desires limes   **poor assimilation**

RELATED REMEDIES
Natrum Mur, Lachesis, Aurum, Causticum
Carcinosin, Golden Spiral

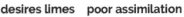

Fluoric Acid
Narcissim

Full name: Fluoricum Acidum
Prepared from distilling Calcium Fluoride in a state of fine powder with Sulphuric Acid.

MENTAL SYMPTOMS:

- Narcissistic
- Materialistic
- Opinionated
- Domineering
- Abuses and reproaches others
- Hurried
- No introspection
- Infantile
- Burning, fiery, sexual energy
- Hypersexual
- Prone to exhaustion as cannot maintain the level of energy they project outwardly
- Selfish - puts self above all else
- Drives people away
- Runs away from responsibilities
- Aversion to own family and sabotages relationships
- Lack of moral code

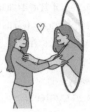

narcissist   domineering

selfish   hypersexual

EVENT THAT CAUSED SYMPTOMS:

- Sexually transmitted disease
- Fluoride poisoning

Fluoric Acid is often used for issues of decay, both physical and emotional. It suits those who feel restless or detached, much like fluoride's ability to erode, helping restore balance where things feel like they're breaking down.

Fluoric Acid
Narcissim

KEYNOTES & PHYSICAL SYMPTOMS:
- Warm blooded
- Bone disorders with deep, slow, decay especially of long bones
- Decay of teeth
- Ulcerations, bedsores, fistulas and varicose veins
- Hair loss
- Chronic headaches
- Prostate issues
- Insomnia
- Water retention and oedema
- Goiter
- Sensation as if a cold wind in eyes
- Degeneration of liver
- Sudden watery discharges from eyes, nose and mouth
- Acrid itchy sweat
- Itching of the orifices
- Hot feet - must uncover them at night

bone issues

decay of teeth

hair loss

oedema

warmth

cold baths

Hindered by:
Heat of room
Warmth
Alcohol
Coffee
Standing

Helped by:
Cool bathing
Open air
Walking
Short sleep
Eating

FOOD:
- Hungry
- Desires spicy foods
- Craving for cold food and water

desires spicy food

craves cold

RELATED REMEDIES
Coffea, Lycopodium, Silica, Syphilinum, Nitric Acid, Sulphur

Golden Spiral
Alignment

MENTAL SYMPTOMS:

- Repairs tired and damaged auras
- Disconnected from source
- Difficulty with transitions
- Helps with letting go - including at the end of life to help aid passing
- Fear of the unknown
- Lacking in purpose
- Past trauma especially surrounding World War 2
- Feeling stuck
- Deep grief
- Difficulty making decisions
- Exhaustion
- Brain fog
- Depression
- Sadness
- Lacking in sense of self

aura repair

disconnected

trauma

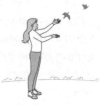

helps to let go

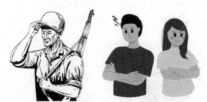

EVENT THAT CAUSED SYMPTOMS:

- Trauma especially issues around World War 2
- Emotional conflicts

The Golden Spiral was proved by the Golden Spiral Proving Collective (founded by Danica Apolline-Matic) in January 2021, involving homeopaths from across the globe, who experienced profound shifts in alignment and expansion during the meditative proving.

Golden Spiral
Alignment

KEYNOTES & PHYSICAL SYMPTOMS:

- Great remedy for general detoxification - supports the liver and improves circulation
- Works at a cellular level to repair DNA and support mitochondrial function
- Sinus issues and congestion
- Aligns and balances the body structurally, especially the spine and skeletal system
- Misaligned teeth
- Autoimmune issues
- Improves respiratory function aiding in breath regulation and clearing congestion
- Low vitality, fatigue and exhaustion
- Brain fog
- Swollen glands
- Difficulty swallowing
- Jaundice
- Stiff joints

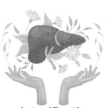
detoxification

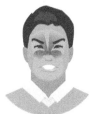
sinusitis

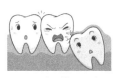
misaligned teeth

supports DNA repair

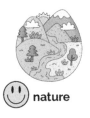
 nature

Hindered by:
N/a

Helped by:
Movement
Warmth
Sunshine
Nature

poor assimilation

FOOD:

- Poor assimilation of food

RELATED REMEDIES
Ayahuasca, Emerald, Spectrum

Hura
'The Black Sheep'

Full name: Hura Brasiliensis
Other names: Assaku Made from the sap of the sandbox tree, known as 'Assaku'. The tree produces a milky latex that is highly toxic and can cause severe irritation.

MENTAL SYMPTOMS:

- Feels like the proverbial 'black sheep'
- Also known as 'the leper's remedy'
- Feels extremely alienated and a primal sense of not belonging, like they live on the edge of society
- Articulate and self depreciating of their history
- May be self loathing
- Believes they are alone in the world
- Delusions that they are despised, feels that they have lost all their friends and that their friends have lost all confidence in them
- Distrust - doesn't know who their real friends are
- Longs for real friends
- Conscientious
- Weeping that alternates with crying
- Irritable
- Depression

'black sheep'

feels alone

distrust

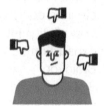

delusions that they are despised

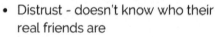

EVENT THAT CAUSED SYMPTOMS:

- Loss of friendship

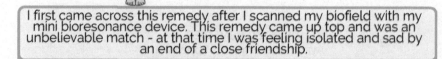

I first came across this remedy after I scanned my biofield with my mini bioresonance device. This remedy came up top and was an unbelievable match - at that time I was feeling isolated and sad by an end of a close friendship.

Hura
'The Black Sheep'

KEYNOTES & PHYSICAL SYMPTOMS:

- This remedy's picture is more on the mental and emotional level. Physical symptoms are more specific as noted below
- Feet and body feel damp
- Lancinating pains
- Colic with diarrhoea and shivering
- Difficult respiration - feeling as if suffocating
- Taste of copper in mouth
- Pimples on face
- Hot flashes
- Sleepiness
- Sensation of a splinter under thumb nails
- Pain behind and in right ear
- Pain in uterus as if compressed or a sharp instrument thrust in it
- Painful lancinations through head
- Sinus issues
- Stiff neck
- Leprosy

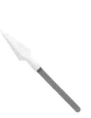

lancinating pains

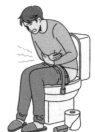

diarrhoea

hot flashes

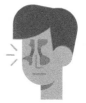

sinus issues

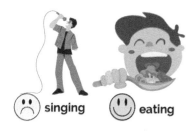

:(**singing**   :) **eating**

Hindered by:
Singing

Helped by:
Eating

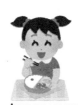

hungry even after eating

FOOD:

- Hungry - sometimes immediately after a meal

RELATED REMEDIES
Anacardium

89

Hyoscyamus
Mania

FULL NAME: Hyoscyamus Niger
Other names: Henbane
Made from the plant Henbane, a member of the Solanaceae (nightshade) family.

MENTAL SYMPTOMS:

- Mania
- Quarrelsome
- Silly and attention seeking - exhibitionist
- Very chatty
- Very jealous
- Anger and rage
- Competitive
- Suspicious
- Pushes the limits and goes too far
- Immature
- Provocative
- Feels abandoned and betrayed
- Vindictive
- Low muttering delirium
- Hallucinations
- Erotic mania
- Wants to be naked
- Fears to eat or drink for fear of being poisoned

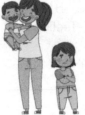

jealousy

silly

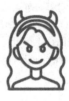

vindictive

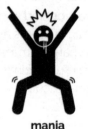

mania

EVENT THAT CAUSED SYMPTOMS:

- Jealousy
- Grief, disappointed love
- Fright
- Suppressed milk

The Solanaceae family of remedies (such as Hyoscamus, Belladonna, Stramonium, Capiscum) are amazing for behavioural issues and have a theme of 'wild but sensitive.'

Hyoscyamus
Mania

KEYNOTES & PHYSICAL SYMPTOMS:

- Restlessness
- Muscle twitches
- Convulsions and trembling
- Epilepsy - sleeps deeply after
- 'Picks at bedclothes'
- Plays with hands
- Dry, hacking, spasmodic cough especially at night
- Toothache especially after being out in cold
- Alcoholism
- Involuntary urination
- Nymphomania
- Exposes genitals
- Hydrophobia
- Toxic gastritis

toothache

convulsions

dry cough

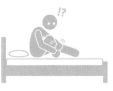
twitching

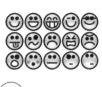
emotions

sitting up

Hindered by:
Emotions
Touch
Cold air
After eating
Evening

Helped by:
Sitting up
Motion
Warmth
Stooping

FOOD:

- Fears to eat or drink from fear of being poisoned
- Aversion to water

fears to eat

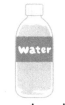
averse to water

RELATED REMEDIES
Belladonna, Stramonium, Lachesis, Tarentula, Anacardium

Lac Caninum
Inferiority

Other name: Dog's milk
Prepared from dog's milk.

MENTAL SYMPTOMS:

- Full of self-loathing
- Extremely self critical
- Submissive and feels inferior
- Despondent
- May cover up low self esteem by wearing make up and being impeccably dressed (similar to Natrum Mur)
- Fears losing control and fear of insanity
- Constant anxiety
- Mood swings and hysteria
- Emotionally intense
- Sensitive to rejection
- Panic attacks
- Suppressed anger
- Fear of fainting and snakes
- May use denial as a coping mechanism
- Useful for grief following the death of a dog

self-loathing despondent

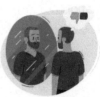

self critical submissive

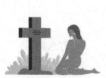

EVENT THAT CAUSED SYMPTOMS:

- Abuse
- Grief

The Lac (or milk) remedies centre around themes of nurturing, identity, belonging, emotional conflict and the struggle between dependence and independence.

Lac Caninum
Inferiority

KEYNOTES & PHYSICAL SYMPTOMS:
- Pains that move from side to side
- Sensitive to touch
- Wandering arthritic pains and rheumatic pains
- Fainting
- Tonsillitis, throat and ear issues that move from side to side
- Swollen and hard stomach
- Stiff neck
- Swollen breasts before menses
- Vertigo as if floating
- Migraines with blurred vision, nausea and vomiting
- Severe, throbbing headaches that may also shift from side to side, often accompanied by visual disturbance
- Fluent nasal discharge often with a sensation of dryness in the nose
- Watery eyes
- Jaw cracks while eating

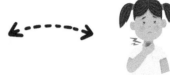

pains that move from side to side   **throat issues**

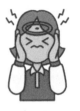 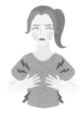

migraines   **swollen breasts**

 touch   **nosebleeds**

Hindered by:
Touch
After sleep
During menses

Helped by:
Cold drinks
Open air
Nosebleeds

FOOD:
- Craves milk but it aggravates

craves milk but it aggravates

> **RELATED REMEDIES**
> Natrum Mur, Thuja, Lachesis, Phosphorus

93

Lac Humanum
Disconnection

Other name: Human breast milk
Prepared from the milk of one nursing mother. This remedy is technically a sarcode but has been included in this section due to its wide scope of action.

MENTAL SYMPTOMS:

- Attachment disorders
- Disconnected - especially from their mother
- Lacks empathy
- Lacks self-esteem and confidence
- Desires approval
- Insecurity and self-doubt as a mother
- Guilt or shame related to motherhood or parenting
- Fastidious and needs order
- Poor concentration
- Feels isolated and lost
- Changeable moods
- Wrings hands
- Averse to company
- Anxiety
- Irritable
- Doesn't want to grow up
- Awkward and clumsy

disconnected

poor bond with mother

insecure

fastidious

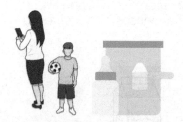

EVENT THAT CAUSED SYMPTOMS:

- Lack of bonding with mother
- Abandonment
- Lack of breastfeeding

While there is overlap, Lac Humanum, made from mature human milk, addresses bonding and abandonment issues, while Lac Maternum, made from the colostrum and milk of nine different mothers, focuses more on birth trauma and initial attachment

Lac Humanum
Disconnection

KEYNOTES & PHYSICAL SYMPTOMS:

- Breastfeeding issues such as sore nipples or mastitis
- Menstrual issues such as heavy bleeding or painful cramps
- Fatigue or exhaustion related to motherhood
- Eating disorders
- Addictions
- Chronic fatigue
- Milk allergies
- Numbness
- Hot flushes
- Cracks in the corners of mouth
- Dry barking cough
- Swollen breasts before menses
- Sensation as if milk is coming into breasts
- Heartburn
- PMS
- Sensation of lump in throat

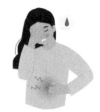

mastitis   PMS

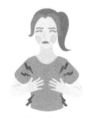

eating   swollen breasts
disorders

Hindered by:
Alcohol
Before menses

Helped by:
Eating
Sex

alcohol   eating

FOOD:

- Desires sweets, starches, chocolate, ginger, bacon, salt
- Aversion to milk, sour foods
- Aggravated by alcohol

desires bacon   aversion to sour foods

> **RELATED REMEDIES**
> Lac Caninum, Anacardium, Phosphorus, Sepia, Pulsatilla

95

Nitric Acid
Pessimism

FULL NAME: Nitricum Acidum
Made from nitric acid, which is a highly corrosive and strong mineral acid with the chemical formula HNO₃.

MENTAL SYMPTOMS:

- The 3 Ps - Pessimistic, pissed off and a pest!
- Vindictive and hateful
- Holds grudges and 'unmoved by apologies'
- Hatred of those who have offended
- Very loyal
- Health anxiety and fear of cancer
- Fear of death
- Irritable especially in the morning
- Headstrong
- Violent anger with fits of rage
- Profane cursing - uses vulgar language
- Discontent
- Everything feels hopeless
- Weak memory
- Confusion

pessimistic

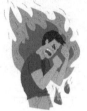

rage

swears and curses

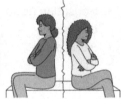

holds grudges

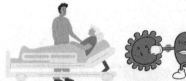

EVENT THAT CAUSED SYMPTOMS:

- Loss of sleep from nursing the sick
- Antibiotics

Known for its ability to burn through almost anything in its material form, Nitric Acid in homeopathy sears through stubborn grudges and deep-seated resentment, bringing relief to both body and soul.

96

Nitric Acid
Pessimism

KEYNOTES & PHYSICAL SYMPTOMS:

- Chilly
- Offensive discharges
- Sticking and splinter-like pains
- Sensation of band around the head and pulsating headache
- Sensitive to noise
- Bloody saliva
- Haemorrhages
- Haemorrhoids that bleed easily
- Anal fissures
- Ringworm
- Cracks at bend of joints
- Eruptions around mouth
- Warts including genital warts
- Ulcers
- Shortness of breath
- Urine smells offensive like horse's urine
- Indigestion and nausea
- Diarrhoea from antibiotics
- Cutting pains after passing stool
- Tonsillitis with cutting pains

haemorrhoids

offensive discharges

splinter-like pains

sensation of band round head

touching

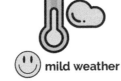
mild weather

Hindered by:
Touching
Jarring
Cold air
Hot weather

Helped by:
Gliding motion
Steady pressure
Mild weather

FOOD:

- Loves fat, herring, salt
- Longs for indigestible things like chalk and earth

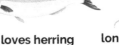
loves herring

longs for chalk

> **RELATED REMEDIES**
> Arsenicum, Merc, Thuja, Lac Caninum, Lachesis, Lycopodium

Oscillococcinum®
The most well-known flu remedy?

OTHER NAME: Anas Barbariae
Prepared from the heart and liver of the Barbary duck, named because under a microscope the cells appear to 'oscillate'.

MENTAL SYMPTOMS:
- Anxiety without a cause
- Impatience
- Likes to be busy
- Stubborn
- Can't bear disorder
- Obsessive
- Fixed ideas
- Fears of dirt and contagion
- Wants to wash hands frequently
- Doesn't want to shake hands in case of germs
- Fears thunderstorms

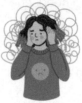

anxiety

fear of germs

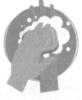

washing hands frequently

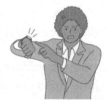

impatience

- Oscillococcinum, a homeopathic flu remedy produced by Boiron Laboratories, is one of the best-selling over-the-counter flu treatments globally, with significant popularity in France.
- For flu symptoms, it is recommended to take at onset and throughout—typically 200c, three times per day or as needed.

In the UK, this remedy is known by its full name as 'Anas Barbariae' - so if ordering from a homeopathic pharmacy look for it under this name rather than Oscillococcinum.

Oscillococcinum®
The most well-known flu remedy?

KEYNOTES & PHYSICAL SYMPTOMS:
- Best-known remedy for flu
- Sensitive to cold
- Sensitive to changes in weather and humidity
- Insomnia - may feel agitated in the night
- Coated white tongue
- Vomiting - even of water
- Bloated stomach
- Diarrhoea
- Pain in appendix
- Blocked nose with catarrh
- Eye catarrh
- Sneezing
- Loss of voice
- Sinus pains
- Pulsating headache at the front of head
- Loss of hearing
- Needle-like pains in ears
- Bronchitis

flu **sensitive to weather changes**

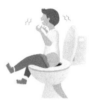 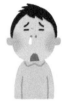

diarrhoea **blocked nose**

 milk   warmth

Hindered by:
Milk
Eggs

Helped by:
Warmth
Rest

 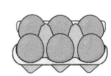

can't digest milk or eggs

FOOD:
- Can't digest milk or eggs

RELATED REMEDIES
Influenzinum, Gelsemium, Arsenicum

Peregrine Falcon
Trapped

Other names: Falco Peregrinus
Prepared from the blood and feather of a captive bred Peregrine Tiercel named Nesbit.

MENTAL SYMPTOMS:

- Desires freedom
- Feels trapped - often by their partner or even their own children
- May do things against instinct for survival
- Feels dominated or controlled
- Intense empathy, especially for the oppressed or vulnerable
- Unpredictable mood swings - sudden outbursts or violent rages
- Swearing
- Internal conflict between yearning for personal freedom and desire to please
- Strong desire for solitude
- Loss of interest in sex
- Compelled to seek truth
- Feels responsible for others
- Difficulty expressing emotions
- Impulsive spending
- Addictions
- Restlessness
- Childlike

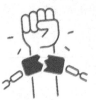

desires freedom

feels trapped

swearing

internal conflict

EVENT THAT CAUSED SYMPTOMS:

- Humiliation
- Confinement or restriction

Proven by Misha Norland and the School of Homeopathy in 1996, Falco Peregrinus is summed up as 'Violent rages of wilfulness in the face of opposition.'

Peregrine Falcon
Trapped

KEYNOTES & PHYSICAL SYMPTOMS:

- Sensation of floating
- Issues with food such as binge eating or severe restrictions
- Photophobia
- Vertigo with nausea
- Headaches with dull pain especially in forehead
- Digestive issues including bloating, flatulence, rumbling and nausea,
- Constipation
- Skin issues including eruptions and dryness
- Trembling or weakness in hands and limbs
- Chest pains
- Dry cough
- Sore throats with mucus
- Mouth ulcers

photophobia

food issues

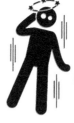
vertigo

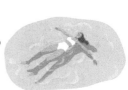
sensation of floating

confinement   **nature**

Hindered by:
Confined spaces
Afternoon
Evening

Helped by:
Open air
Nature
Movement

FOOD:

- Craves chocolate, sweets
- Desire for beer, pickles
- Aversion to tomatoes, cucumbers
- Appetite fluctuates (hungry or no desire)

desires beer

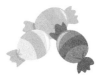
craves sweets

RELATED REMEDIES
Anacardium, Lac Caninum, Natrum Mur, Platina, Thuja

Placenta
Isolation

Full name: Placenta Humana
Prepared from human placenta. This remedy is technically a sarcode but has been included in this section due to its wide scope of action.

MENTAL SYMPTOMS:
- Feels unloved, isolated and misunderstood
- Separation
- Rebellious
- Anger with family
- Resentment and regret
- Overwhelm
- Exhaustion
- Doesn't see any future
- Scared of everything
- Fear of failure, being late and closed spaces
- Anxiety and panic attacks
- Emotional instability
- Irritability
- Nostalgia with flashbacks
- Attracted to the colour burgundy
- Dreams of babies
- Delusion is pregnant
- Grief

isolated

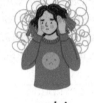
anxiety

nostalgia

unloved

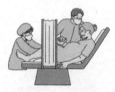

EVENT THAT CAUSED SYMPTOMS:
- Birth trauma
- Fear during pregnancy, especially about the baby's health
- Bad news

In 1999, the Welsh School of Homeopathy conducted a proving of the remedy Placenta in a 40c potency, representing the 40 weeks of pregnancy.

Placenta
Isolation

KEYNOTES & PHYSICAL SYMPTOMS:

- Constriction and pressure
- Heart palpitations
- Head pressure
- Pins and needles
- Pressure on chest
- Bloated and tender stomach
- Flatulence
- Sleepy - likes catnaps
- Symptoms appear around menses and ovulation
- Irregular periods
- Infertility
- Placenta previa or weak placenta
- Chilly and craves warmth
- Insomnia
- Babies who refuse breast milk
- 'Blue' babies
- Eating disorders
- Allergies
- High sexual energy

head pressure　**constriction**

pins and needles　**sleepy**

 cold　 **warmth**

Hindered by:
Cold
Hormones

Helped by:
Warmth
Massage

FOOD:

- Lack of thirst and appetite
- Desires spicy food, sweets, chocolate
- Aversion to nuts

 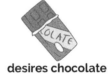

desires spice　**desires chocolate**

> **RELATED REMEDIES**
> Carcinosin, Lycopodium, Pulsatilla, Sepia

Platina
Superiority

Full name: Platinum Metallicum
Prepared from the precious metal Platinum.

MENTAL SYMPTOMS:
- Delusions of grandeur
- Haughty, narcissitic and self absorbed
- Contempt for others
- Arrogant
- Megalomania
- Wounded pride
- Fault finding
- Feels they have no place in the world and doesn't belong even with family
- Delusion that people are devils and the enemy
- Violent impulses
- Changeable mood
- Hysteria before menses
- Hypersexual and nymphomania
- Alternating physical and mental symptoms
- Discontented and sad
- Argumentative and abrupt
- Anxious

delusions of grandeur   arrogant

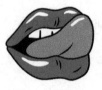
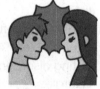

nymphomania   argumentative

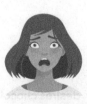
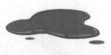

EVENT THAT CAUSED SYMPTOMS:
- Fright, bereavement
- Sexual excess
- Haemorrhages

> The Platina individual rarely has enough self-awareness to recognise the Platina traits in themselves, often instead referring to everyone else around them as having those traits that they themselves have.

Platina
Superiority

KEYNOTES & PHYSICAL SYMPTOMS:
- Constricted or bandaged sensation
- Numbness and coldness
- Spasms and cramping
- Affinity to sexual organs
- Sexual mania
- Vaginismus - sex is impossible
- Haemorrhages with black clots
- Colic from lead poisoning
- Painfully sensitive genitals
- Dark clotted menses
- Headaches with squeezing cramps
- Sensation of constriction in stomach
- Constipation when travelling
- Tapeworms
- Lost sense of proportion in vision - objects appear smaller than what they are

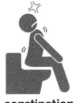

constipation when travelling

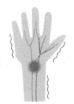

numbness

vaginismus

spasms

 emotions **stretching**

Hindered by:
Emotions
Sex
During menses
Touch
Evening

Helped by:
Walking in open air
Sunshine
Stretching
Motion

FOOD:
- Ravenous hunger with hasty eating
- Loss of appetite when sad

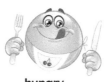

hungry

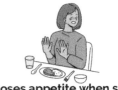

loses appetite when sad

RELATED REMEDIES
Sepia, Nux Vomica

Plutonium
Destruction

FULL NAME: Plutonium Nitricum
A small, non-radioactive sample of plutonium was succussed and diluted to create the homeopathic remedy.

MENTAL SYMPTOMS:

- Plutonium's core conflict: The urge to express immense power and energy versus the intense fear of its consequences, leading to a cold, detached existence - 'essence of me' has gone
- Inner light feels unreachable
- Profound loneliness, isolation and separation
- Serious with too many responsibilities
- Philosophical or religious thoughts
- Leaves body easily
- No compassion - acts automatically and coldly
- Violent outbursts, aggression and dominant behaviour
- Fear of one's own impulses
- Depressed
- Health anxiety
- Claustrophobia
- Sensation of existential threat
- Useful for shock and trauma when other remedies fail to act

detachment

isolation

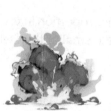

fears
impulses

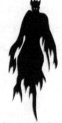

inner light
gone

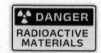

EVENT THAT CAUSED SYMPTOMS:
- Radiation

DREAMS:

- Dreams of passively watching from above but acts when the dream repeats
- Fallen angels, lost paradise and bats hanging upside down

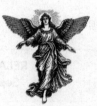

Plutonium
Destruction

KEYNOTES & PHYSICAL SYMPTOMS:
- Periodical fatigue
- Useful for treating the individual with serious pathologies such as those with bone cancer, lung cancer, brain tumours, leukemia, Hodgkin's diseases, AIDS

| periodical fatigue | serious pathologies |

- Genetic defects, congenital diseases
- Radiation poisoning
- Sensitive to EMFs
- Sensitive to light, especially blue lights
- Feels burning, heaviness, crushing weight

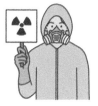

| radiation poisoning | blue light sensitivity |

- Headache, forehead, shattering
- Eyes burning
- Enlarged thyroid
- Lung complaints: fibrosis, narrowing of the blood vessels
- Vomiting and/or diarrhoea
- Bone marrow affections

 night   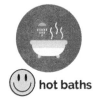 hot baths

Hindered by:
Night
Sunset
3pm
Overcast weather
Walking

Helped by:
Hot applications
Hot baths
Long sleep
Massage

FOOD:
- Desires bacon, raw meat, lamb, pork, ham, fat

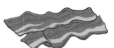

desires bacon and raw meat

RELATED REMEDIES
Aurum, Carcinosin, Medhorrinum, Rad Brom,
Stramonium, Syphilinum, Tarentula, X-Ray

Rad Brom
Fear of the dark

FULL NAME: Radium Bromatum
Made from the radioative element radium combined with bromine.

MENTAL SYMPTOMS:
- Guilt over surviving when others did not
- Anxiety and restlessness, particularly at night, with a feeling of impending doom or that something 'terrible' will happen
- Fear of the dark
- Fear of being alone
- Wants someone with them all the time
- Profound sadness or depression, often with a sense of hopelessness or despair
- Apprehensive
- Fear of death, radiation or contamination
- Health anxiety with fear of developing serious illnesses
- Tired, lack of motivation

fear of the dark

fear of being alone

apprehensive

tired

EVENT THAT CAUSED SYMPTOMS:
- Radiation
- X-Ray
- Burns

In its material form, Rad Brom is a luminous salt that causes the air surrounding it, even when encased in a tube, to glow a brilliant green.

Rad Brom
Fear of the dark

KEYNOTES & PHYSICAL SYMPTOMS:

- Issues with skin and nerves
- Severe aching pains all over which is helped by moving about
- Shifting pains
- Numbness
- Dry burning heat throughout body - craves cool air
- Electric shocks through the body during sleep
- Radiation burns and ulcers
- Chronic rheumatic arthritis
- Backache between shoulders and lumbar-sacral region
- Pain in toes
- Itching all over body
- Eczema after X-Rays
- Acne rosacea
- Chest feels constricted
- Air hunger

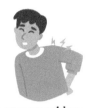

severe aching   **burning**

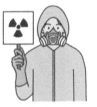 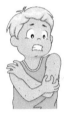

radiation burns   **itching**

 shaving   motion

Hindered by:
Smoking
Shaving
Washing
Night
Warmth of bed

Helped by:
Lying down
After sleep
Motion
Hot bath

FOOD:
- Craves pork
- Averse to sweets

craves pork   **averse to sweets**

RELATED REMEDIES
Anacardium, X-Ray, Rhus Tox, Causticum

Saccharum
Sugar as a substitute for love

> **FULL NAME: Saccharum Officinale**
> Prepared from the fresh stem of the sugar cane.

MENTAL SYMPTOMS:
- Lack of self love
- Fear of abandonment, especially of mother's love
- Desperate for love
- Feels alone
- Antisocial
- Needs cuddles
- Fear of failure
- Jealousy, especially of siblings
- Homesickness
- Talkative
- Restlessness
- Mood swings
- Plays antics
- Aggression and fits of anger
- 'Hanger' - irritable before breakfast or when hungry
- Difficulty concentrating
- Feeling the need to acquire new things
- Dissatisfaction

lack of self love

fear of abandonment

fits of anger

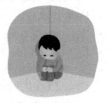

feels alone

EVENT THAT CAUSED SYMPTOMS:
- Being rewarded by sweets rather than love
- Lack of affection

> Whilst Saccharum is most frequently prescribed as a constitutional remedy, it is sometimes prescribed by homeopaths in a low potency to support gut health, where the symptoms fit.

Saccharum
Sugar as a substitute for love

KEYNOTES & PHYSICAL SYMPTOMS:

- Lack of self love
- Sugar addictions
- Sensitive to pain or feels no pain at all
- Fainting from pain
- Hypoglycaemia
- Early morning waking
- Dryness of skin, hair, mouth or stool
- General gut issues
- Great appetite but often emaciated
- Acidity and indigestion
- Anal itching and/or worms
- Candida or white coating on tongue
- Nail biting in children or smoking in adults
- Stomach pains or pain in the spleen
- Painful ovulation
- Hot lower limbs which must be uncovered
- Hyperactivity
- Developmental delays

lack of pain

early waking

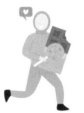
sugar addictions

gut issues

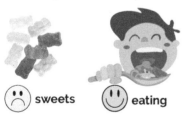
sweets   eating

Hindered by:
Excitement
Sweets
Chocolate
Warm weather

Helped by:
Evening
Eating

FOOD:

- Desires chocolate, sweets, licorice, meat, tea, milk
- Thirsty for large amounts of water or tea

craves chocolate

thirsty

RELATED REMEDIES
Belladonna, Calc Carb, Stramonium, Lachesis, Lycopodium, Opium, Carcinosin

111

Sanguinaria
Burning intensity

FULL NAME: Sanguinaria Canadensis
Other name: Blood-root
Prepared from the fresh root of the Blood-root, a perennial, herbaceous flowering plant native to eastern North America.

MENTAL SYMPTOMS:

- Feels confident of recovery (unlike many remedies which more frequently have a despair of recovery)
- Confused mind
- Feels better by belching
- Anxiety
- Dread before vomiting
- Grumbling
- Angry
- Sensitive to insults - may get in a rage
- Sensitive to noise
- Morose
- Sleepiness
- Doesn't want to move or make any effort
- Sensation as if paralysed when lying on back

confident of recovery

confused

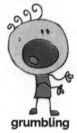

grumbling

better for belching

EVENT THAT CAUSED SYMPTOMS:

- Menopause
- Emotional stress

I personally found relief from persistent migraines with Sanguinaria, where the headaches began at the back of the head, moved to the right eye, and worsened in sunlight—a textbook case reflecting the remedy's characteristic symptom picture

Sanguinaria
Burning intensity

KEYNOTES & PHYSICAL SYMPTOMS:
- Burning heat and sensations
- Right sided
- Feels sick and faint from smell of flowers
- Periodical headaches
- Headaches and migraines that ascend from occiput to over right eye
- Vomiting with headaches
- Flashes with migraines
- Burning palms and soles
- Hot flushes
- Pneumonia
- Hayfever
- Rust-coloured sputum
- Polyps, growths and tumours
- Biliousness
- Shoulder pains
- Rheumatism

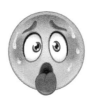
hot flushes

migraines with flashes

right sided

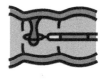
polyps

 sweets

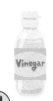 **sour things**

Hindered by:
Touch
Sweets
Menopause

Helped by:
Sour things
Vomiting
Cool air
Darkness
Belching

FOOD:
- Loss of appetite
- Unquenchable thirst
- Aversion to butter
- Sweet things aggravate

averse to butter

thirsty

RELATED REMEDIES
Ant Tart, Phosphorus, Belladonna,
Morgan Gaertner

Scorpion
Survival

FULL NAME: Androctonus Amurreuxi
Prepared from the African fat-tailed scorpion which lives in North Africa, Mali and Asia.

MENTAL SYMPTOMS:
- Survivor
- Intense
- Desires to control
- Antisocial loner
- Charismatic and magnetic
- History of violence or cruelty
- Intelligent and manipulative
- Sexually aware from a young age
- Irritable
- Curses and swears
- Violent - capacity to kill
- No remorse after an argument
- Feels disconnected from the world
- Rebellious
- Extreme and changeable moods
- Paranoia, panic attacks and fear
- Impatient
- Delusions someone is plotting against them

survivor   charismatic

violent   paranoia

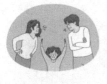

EVENT THAT CAUSED SYMPTOMS:
- Violence
- Fright

DREAMS:
- Oppressive dreams
- Dreams of being murdered, attacked, heads being chopped off, toilets, climbing ladders, jealousy

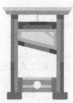 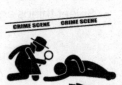

Scorpion
Survival

KEYNOTES & PHYSICAL SYMPTOMS:
- Desires fresh air
- Anxiety in heart and chest area
- Anxiety in stomach
- Hypersensitive to light and noise - will keep curtains closed
- Wears sunglasses - doesn't want to be seen
- Strabismus
- Dilated pupils
- Menopausal panic attacks with palpitations
- Early and short menses
- Backache
- Nightmares
- Fatigue
- Headaches from the sun
- Copious saliva
- Sweating at night and in the morning

photophobia   **anxiety in chest**

 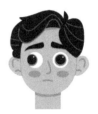

nightmares   **strabismus**

Hindered by:
Sun

Helped by:
Milk

sun   milk

FOOD:
- Eats little and often
- Extreme thirst
- Aversion to courgettes
- Craves chocolate

thirsty   **averse to courgettes**

> **RELATED REMEDIES**
> Anarcadium, Tarentula, Syphilinum

115

Shungite - Carbon C60
Purification

 Prepared from a piece of 'noble' shungite, a rare, carbon-rich mineral found primarily in the Karelia region of Russia, known for its purported protective and healing properties.

MENTAL SYMPTOMS:
- Brings buried issues to the surface
- Causes hidden forces, including miasms, to reveal themselves
- Unresolved or suppressed traumas which may have been hidden for personal or karmic reasons
- Lack of awareness
- Sense of being 'switched off'
- Inattentiveness
- Emotional dullness
- Irritability
- Profound lack of motivation
- Sees but does not perceive
- Addicted to energies or substances which may stimulate or dull the senses
- Ungrounded

unresolved issues   **unaware**

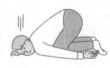

irritable   **unmotivated**

EVENT THAT CAUSED SYMPTOMS:
- Fluoride
- Radiation
- Toxins
- Dental work

Shungite is one of the 'new' remedies which was first proved by the Guild of Homeopaths in 2017.

Shungite - Carbon C60
Purification

KEYNOTES & PHYSICAL SYMPTOMS:

- Clears deep, hidden toxicities
- Rebalances endocrine system
- Fluoride poisoning - confusion, insomnia, throat irritation
- Heavy metal accumulation - muscular weakness, nerve issues
- Candida overgrowth - digestive imbalance, mental fog
- Radiation exposure - fatigue, mental dullness, skin reaction
- Drug or medication induced imbalances such as heightened sensitivity, eczema, asthma, digestive conditions or unexplained fatigue
- 'Post-viral fatigue'
- Lingering coughs
- Persistent parasites
- Tooth decay
- Nasal congestion

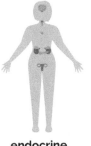

endocrine system issues

toxicities

lingering coughs

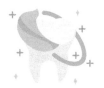

fluoride issues

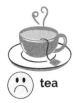

tea

Hindered by:
Suppression
Any toxins
Tea

Helped by:
N/a

FOOD:

- Cravings for addictive acidic substances that contribute to obesity

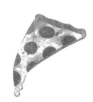

desires addictive acidic foods

> **RELATED REMEDIES**
> Calc Carb, Thuja

Sol
Never been well since sunburn

Other name: Sunlight
Prepared by exposing lactose to concentrated sunray.

MENTAL SYMPTOMS:
- Decisive
- Assertive
- Impatient to make decisions
- Mental restlessness
- Wants to be healthy - has the urge to eat lots of fruit
- Light headed
- Disorientated
- Depression
- Sensitive
- Suspicious
- Desires to bang head and scream
- Wants to escape
- Anxiety, nervousness and trembling
- Delusion of being pursued
- Anxiety of people coming towards them

decisive

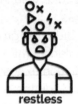
restless

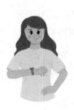

impatient

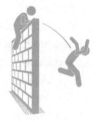
escapism

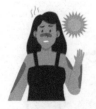

EVENT THAT CAUSED SYMPTOMS:
- Sunburn
- Radiation

Sol is considered an imponderable remedy because it is derived from an intangible source — the pure energy of sunlight — capturing its vibrational essence without any material substance, much like other imponderables such as X-Ray.

Sol
Never been well since sunburn

KEYNOTES & PHYSICAL SYMPTOMS:

- Very sensitive to the sun
- Chronic sun headaches
- Photophobia
- Painful eyes from glare of the sun
- Sunburns easily
- Moles, growths and sunspots
- Cataracts
- Hands and feet are cold
- Very cold - chilled to the bone
- Shivering
- Sensation as if weight on chest
- Backaches
- Lupus
- Trembling in heart
- Faintness
- Anxiety in stomach

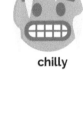

sensitive to sun   **skin issues**

chilly   **photophobia**

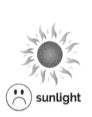 sunlight    hot bath

Hindered by:
Sunlight
Standing

Helped by:
Hot baths
Short naps
Cloudy weather

FOOD:

- Desires hot chocolate, oranges, refreshing things, meat, lime juice, cheese, salty foods

desires oranges   **desires meat**

RELATED REMEDIES
X-Ray, Natrum Mur

119

Spectrum
Flow

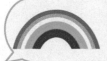

Other name: Rainbow
Prepared by exposing ethanol to the rays of the sun shining through a prism.

MENTAL SYMPTOMS:

- Fear of change
- Apprehension
- Ungrounded and spaced out
- Poor intuition
- Depression - inability to see the way forward
- Depressive states brought on by drugs
- Lacks mental clarity
- Mental breakdown
- Moody teenagers
- Needs structure
- Mood disturbances relating to menopause
- Stressed after hard work
- Fearfulness
- Confusion

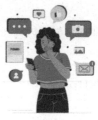

fears change

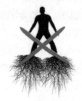

ungrounded

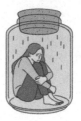

depression

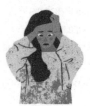

mental breakdown

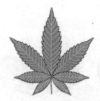

EVENT THAT CAUSED SYMPTOMS:

- Recreational drugs
- Nicotine poisoning

This remedy is 'most frequently used as an intercurrent or when indicated remedies fail (this is particularly true after psoric and constitutional remedies) or as the 'glue' between other indicated remedies in conditions that call for detoxing.' Griffith

Spectrum
Flow

KEYNOTES & PHYSICAL SYMPTOMS:

- Encourages flow of bodily fluids
- Releases meridian blockages
- Toxic overload
- Hot flushes
- Fever with night sweats
- Sensations of trickling water
- Blood clots
- Oedema
- Skin issues such as psoriasis and eczema
- Headache with burning pain
- Watery left eye
- Conjunctivitis of left then right eye
- Photophobia
- High cholesterol
- High blood presure

encourages flow

toxicity

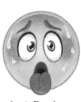

hot flushes

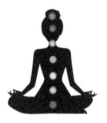

meridian blockages

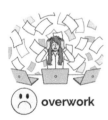

overwork

structure

Hindered by:
Overwork

Helped by:
Structure

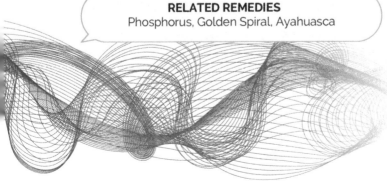

RELATED REMEDIES
Phosphorus, Golden Spiral, Ayahuasca

Tarentula
Restlessness

FULL NAME: Tarentula Hispanica
Other name: Wolf Spider, Spanish Tarantula
Prepared from the Tarentula spider.

MENTAL SYMPTOMS:
- Extremely restless and hurried
- Hyperactive behaviour and a tendency to fidget
- Nervousness and hysteria
- Obstinate
- Mania and erratic moods
- Destructive impulses
- Desires the presence of people yet averse to company
- Cunning and sly
- Impulsiveness and a lack of self-control
- Intense
- Tormenting behaviour
- Ungrateful
- Anxious
- Sensation of being small
- Loves music and dancing
- Sensitivity to noise
- May fake fainting

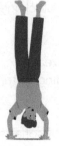
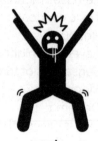

restless   mania

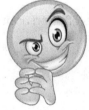

cunning   loves music

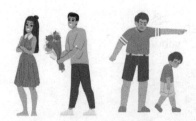

EVENT THAT CAUSED SYMPTOMS:
- Unrequited love
- Bad news
- Punishment

This was the first remedy that I ever administered as a paper remedy (see p21). My homeopath suggested doing so as I did not have the physical remedy to hand. I was sceptical but amazed at the result!

Tarentula
Restlessness

KEYNOTES & PHYSICAL SYMPTOMS:

- Symptoms appear suddenly
- Nervous disorders
- Violent pains 'as if thousands of needles were pricking' (Phatak)
- Can aid agony of death pains
- Sensation of constriction
- Attacks of suffocation
- Painfully sensitive spine
- Sepsis
- Purplish skin
- Painful boils with burning sensation
- Tremors, twitches and jerking
- Restless legs
- Multiple sclerosis with trembling
- Rapid heartbeat
- Itching of the vulva (Pruritus vulvae) especially after menses
- Insomnia before midnight

suddeness

painful boils

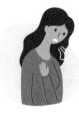

suffocation attacks

violent pains

touch

music

Hindered by:
Periodicity
Touch
Cold
Damp
After menses

Helped by:
Music
Rubbing
Sweating
Exertion
Open air

FOOD:

- Craving for sand, raw food and salt
- Aversion to meat
- Thirsty for cold water
- Refuses food

craves sand

averse to meat

> **RELATED REMEDIES**
> Similar to Arsenicum - if Arsenicum seems indicated
> but fails to act then give Tarentula.

Umbilical Cord
Cut off

Full name: Umbilicus Humanus
Prepared from human umbilical cord. This remedy is technically a sarcode but has been included in this section due to its wide scope of action.

MENTAL SYMPTOMS:

- Shock and trauma
- Difficulty with boundaries
- Feeling cut off, disconnected or isolated from others
- Feels like the outsider
- Fear of rejection or abandonment
- Clingy
- Attachment issues
- Unhealthy ties
- Self-reproach
- Feels the victim
- Sleep issues - may wake feeling paralysed
- Confused identity
- Hates anything around the neck
- Times feel distorted

confused identity

feels cut off

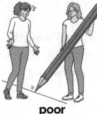

poor boundaries

clingy

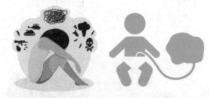

EVENT THAT CAUSED SYMPTOMS:

- Birth trauma, especially complications involving the umbilical cord such as cord around the neck

DREAMS:

- Dreams of death
- Dreams of violence - being cut or stabbed, hanging
- Dreams of wounded or lost children

MISSING

Umbilical Cord
Cut off

KEYNOTES & PHYSICAL SYMPTOMS:

- General right sided issues
- Joint pain or stiffness
- Issues related to circulation especially poor peripheral circulation or cold extremities
- Reproductive issues such as infertility or painful periods
- Sensation of glass in throat
- Menopause issues
- Umbilical hernia
- Symptoms of digestive issues, particularly in the navel area (pain, cramping or discomfort around the umbilicus)
- Gas and bloating
- Painful scars
- Scar tissues
- Birth related trauma
- Fatigue and weakness

joint pain   right sided

 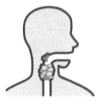

stomach issues   sensation of glass in throat

 cold

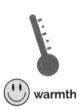 warmth

Hindered by: Cold

Helped by: Warmth

FOOD:

- Craves sweets, chocolate
- Aversion to spicy foods

 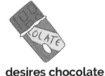

averse to spice   desires chocolate

> **RELATED REMEDIES**
> Lac Humanum, Placenta, Carcinosin, Pulsatilla

Veratrum
Delusional

FULL NAME: Veratrum Album
Other names: White Hellebore Made from a highly toxic perennial plant of the Liliaceae family, which contains powerful alkaloids.

MENTAL SYMPTOMS:

- Religious insanity
- Despairs of their salvation
- Delusions of impending doom
- Violent delirium
- Mania with desire to cut and tear things
- Anguish with fear of death
- Deceitful
- Feels unlucky
- Curses and shrieks
- Sings, whistles and laughs
- Runs from place to place
- Imagines herself pregnant
- Melancholy
- Indifference
- Sullen
- Broods in silence
- Haughtiness
- Hyperactive and disobedient children
- Critical

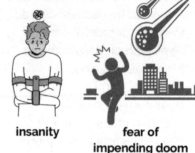

insanity   fear of
              impending doom

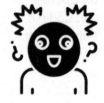

sullen   mania

EVENT THAT CAUSED SYMPTOMS:

- Post-operative shock
- Suppressed rashes
- Fright

Lemke states 'the overmentalized state in Veratrum tends to create paranoid delusions that people are out to get them or that there is a mass conspiracy, making it useful as a remedy for schizophrenia.'

Veratrum
Delusional

KEYNOTES & PHYSICAL SYMPTOMS:

- Internal cold - cold sweat and cold skin
- Profuse evacuations - stools, vomit, sweat, urine
- Progressive weakness
- Collapse with weakness
- Thirsty for cold water which is vomited
- Hungry despite nausea
- Chronic vomiting - projectile vomit or vomits froth
- Cold feeling in stomach
- Colic as if bowels in knots
- As if hot coals in abdomen
- Fainting
- Pale blue face
- Cramps in calves
- Tip of nose ice cold
- Large stools forcibly evacuated
- Cholera

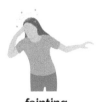 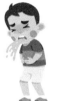

fainting   vomiting

cold sweat   pale blue face

drinking   warmth

Hindered by:
Drinking
Exertion
Wet weather
Before and
during menses

Helped by:
Warmth
Hot drinks
Eating
Lying

FOOD:

- Craves ice water, salt, lemon, sour fruit
- Aggravated by fruits, potatoes, green vegetables

craves ice water   fruit aggravates

RELATED REMEDIES
Belladonna, Stramonium, Tuberculinum, Medhorrinum

Vernix
Need for protection

Full name: Vernix Caseosa Prepared from human vernix, the waxy coating that develops around 17-20 weeks of gestation. This remedy is technically a sarcode but has been included in this section due to its wide scope of action.

MENTAL SYMPTOMS:

- Enables connection with the outside world without feeling overwhelmed by it
- Becomes overly involved with others - lacks boundaries
- Lack of protection
- Insecure and clingy
- OCD
- Rituals
- Hoarder
- Hopelessness
- Sensory processing issues
- Hypersensitive to emotions and external stimuli
- Lacks own identity
- Feels guilty
- Sees themselves as a victim
- Fantasises

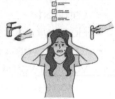

lack of protection

OCD

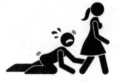

insecurity

hopelessness

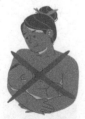
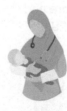

EVENT THAT CAUSED SYMPTOMS:

- Traumatic, fast births
- Lack of skin contact after birth

Matridonal remedies (including Amniotic Fluid, Placenta, Vernix, Umbilical Cord, Lac Humanum) are homeopathic remedies derived from substances related to conception, pregnancy and birth, focusing on nurturing, connection and healing birth-related trauma.

Vernix
Need for protection

KEYNOTES & PHYSICAL SYMPTOMS:

- Skin conditions - dryness, peeling or a need for hydration, mirroring the protective function of vernix on a newborn's skin
- Eczema in babies with no clear cause
- Sleeplessness
- Respiratory issues such as restriction which may be linked to birth trauma
- Hypersensitivity to environmental factors like cold air, wind or pollutants
- Weak terrain, frequent acute issues in children.
- Digestive discomfort, especially in newborns or infants, such as colic, regurgitation or difficulty digesting milk

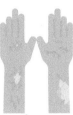
dry or peeling skin

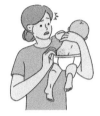
eczema in newborns

sleeplessness

hypersensitivity

cold

warmth

Hindered by: Cold

Helped by: Warmth

FOOD:

- Averse to dry foods
- Craves comfort foods like porridge

averse dry food

craves comfort food

> **RELATED REMEDIES**
> Phosphorus, Carcinosin, Stramonium, Opium, X-Ray, Spongia

X-Ray
Low vitality

 Made via exposing liquid to x-rays through a glass bottle, then subjecting to the usual dilution and succussion process.

MENTAL SYMPTOMS:

- Aversion to company
- Delusions of seeing fire
- Intense irritability
- Sudden desire to kill especially before and during menses
- Depression, sadness, melancholy
- Suicidal thoughts, with impulses to throw oneself from a height
- Tendency to uncover hidden truths
- Feeling invisible or 'seeing through walls' like a sense of having x-ray vision
- Desire for control
- Weak memory
- Sleepy
- Fear of tunnels

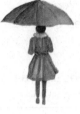

aversion to company

sadness

desire to kill before menses

suicidal thoughts

EVENT THAT CAUSED SYMPTOMS:

- Radiation
- X-Ray

Homeopathic X-Ray was developed after the discovery of x-rays and has been used to treat various vague, deep-seated conditions and radiation exposure, reflecting its ability to bring hidden issues to the surface both physically and emotionally.

X-Ray
Low vitality

KEYNOTES & PHYSICAL SYMPTOMS:

- Rouses vital force so that suppressed symptoms are brought to the surface
- Vague symptoms only
- Chronic fatigue with nausea
- Low vitality
- Anaemia
- Night sweats
- Suitable for vague, deep-seated symptoms or illnesses with a tendency toward malignancy
- Conditions following repeated x-rays, especially in childhood
- Obstinate skin diseases, wounds and ulcers that fail to heal.
- Sterility or impotence without a clear cause
- Warty growths

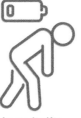

low vitality

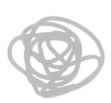

vague symptoms

warts

slow healing wounds

 cold

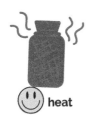 heat

Hindered by:
Cold, open air
Movement
Afternoon, evening and night
When in bed

Helped by:
Hot applications

FOOD:

- Anorexia
- Desires sweets

anorexia

desires sweets

> **RELATED REMEDIES**
> Carcinosin, Phosphorus, Secale

Miasms

The next section provides an overview of the miasms in the same familiar format shown previously:
- Psoric Miasm
- Syphilitic Miasm
- Sycotic Miasm
- Tubercular Miasm
- Cancer Miasm
- A new Strep Miasm?

Psoric Miasm
Deficiency and under-functioning

 The homeopathic remedy which is used to treat the Psoric miasm is called PSORINUM and it is a nosode made from Scabies.

MENTAL PRESENTATION
- Concerned with most basic survival
- People who are only just managing
- Sense of lack
- Poverty consciousness
- Anxiety especially around health, business or money
- Fear of death, cancer, poverty, future, failure
- Feels separated from source
- Hopelessness about the future
- Suicidal thoughts
- Despair of recovery
- Weak memory
- Sense of foreboding
- Feels unusually well before an illness

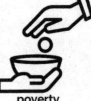

lack

poverty consciousness

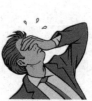
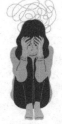

despair of recovery

hopeless

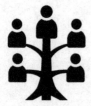
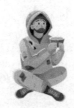

EVENT THAT CAUSED SYMPTOMS:
- Inherited miasm from ancestor
- Poor hygiene and diet

DREAMS:
- Anxious dreams
- Sexual dreams

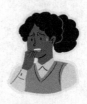

134

Psoric Miasm
Deficiency and under-functioning

KEYNOTES & PHYSICAL SYMPTOMS:

- Under-functioning
- Offensive discharges and eruptions
- Skin issues with itching that 'leads to despair' and scratches until bleeds
- Allergies and hayfever
- Lack of vitality and reaction - Psorinum can boost the vital force
- Frequent acute illnesses
- Very chilly - wants warm clothes and hates drafts
- Malnutrition
- May be constipated or have loose stools
- Feels hungry with tendency towards hypoglycaemia
- Parasites, lice or scabies
- Perspires at night
- Eruptions in folds of joints

Under-functioning   **offensive discharges**

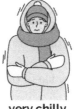 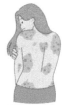

very chilly   **skin issues**

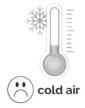 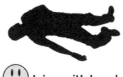

cold air   **lying with head low**

Hindered by:
Cold, open air
From suppressions
Before thunderstorms
Fasting

Helped by:
Lying with head low
Heat
Warm clothing
Sweating

FOOD:

- Ravenous with extreme hunger before illness
- Desires beer
- Averse to pork

 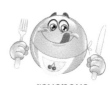

desires beer   **ravenous**

> **RELATED REMEDIES**
> Sulphur, Calc Carb, Lycopodium

Sycotic Miasm
Excess

 The homeopathic remedy which is used to treat the Sycotic miasm is called MEDORRHINUM and it is a nosode made from Gonorrhoea.

MENTAL PRESENTATION

- Excess!
- Lots of energy - passionate with enormous appetite for life
- Impulsive, unstable and inconsistent
- Hurried and anxious
- Time passes too slowly
- Hyperactivity in children
- Panic attacks
- Life feels unreal, like a dream
- Disconnected
- Sex, drugs and rock and roll - party animals, alcoholism, drug abuse
- Surge of energy in the evening
- Loves animals or extremely cruel to them
- Shuns responsibilities
- Fears the dark, monsters and feels as if someone is behind her
- Weak memory
- Clairvoyance

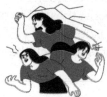

excess energy

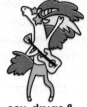

sex, drugs & music

dreamy

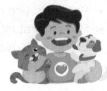

loves animals

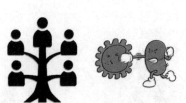

EVENT THAT CAUSED SYMPTOMS:
- Inherited miasm from ancestor
- Suppressed gonorrhoea

DREAMS:
- Of monsters
- Of dead people

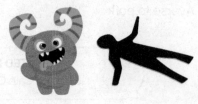

Sycotic Miasm
Excess

KEYNOTES & PHYSICAL SYMPTOMS:

- Overproduction
- Skin issues relating to overgrowths - warts, cysts, polyps, fibroids
- Chronic sinusitis and/or rhinitis
- Chronic throat clearing
- Peptic ulcers which wake at 2am
- Genital issues including cysts and fibroids
- Infertility
- Excessive sexual energy
- Urinary issues - chronic cystitis
- Nighttime bedwetting
- Kidney issues including colic
- Benign tumours
- Glue ear
- Asthma
- Rheumatism
- Sleep with bum in the air in the knee/chest position
- Bites nails
- Hot feet

Over-production

overgrowths

knee/chest sleep position

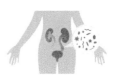

genito-urinary issues

 damp

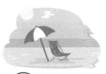

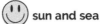 **sun and sea**

Hindered by:
Damp
Sunrise to sunset
3am-4am
When thinking of issues

Helped by:
The seashore
Sunshine
Nighttime
Lying on tummy

FOOD:

- Craving for ice, green fruits, oranges, meat, fat
- Aversion to aubergine and 'slimy' foods

averse to aubergines

craves oranges

> **RELATED REMEDIES**
> Thuja, Pulsatilla

Syphylitic Miasm
Self-destruction

The homeopathic remedy which is used to treat the Syphylitic miasm is called SYPHILINUM and it is a nosode made from Treponema pallidum spirochaete bacterium.

MENTAL PRESENTATION

- Destructive - as if they have a deathwish
- Insane or feels as if going insane
- Fear of germs
- Fastidious and compulsive checking
- OCD and excessive handwashing
- Suicidal depression
- Creative genius
- Anti-social
- Depression especially in winter
- Loss of memory
- Nervy and on edge
- Angry or irritable
- Addictions including alcoholism
- Despair of recovery and feels hopeless
- Hypochondria and health anxiety
- Fears the night
- Prone to 'accidents'

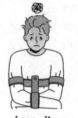
insanity

self-destructive

suicidal

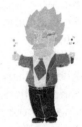
creative genius

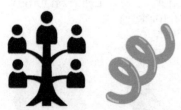

EVENT THAT CAUSED SYMPTOMS:

- Inherited miasm from ancestor
- Syphilis in one's own lifetime

DREAMS:

- Disconnected dreams
- Dreams of diseases

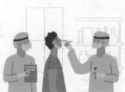

Syphylitic Miasm
Self-destruction

KEYNOTES & PHYSICAL SYMPTOMS:

- Suicide
- 'Accidents'
- Central nervous system issues such as Multiple Sclerosis, ALS
- Bone pain and issues including abscesses
- Burning pains
- Mucus membrane issues such as ulcers, abscesses, fistulas
- Nightsweats
- Intense pain at night
- Eczema which itches at night
- Hair loss
- Tooth decay
- Severe insomnia
- Pale, wrinkled skin
- Excessive saliva especially when sleeping
- Headache in bones of head

accidents

central nervous system issues

bone issues

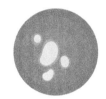
ulcers, abscesses

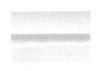
seaside

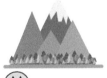
mountains

Hindered by:
Nighttime
Seaside
Full moon

Helped by:
Mountains
During the day
Heat
Slow motion

FOOD:

- Craves alcohol
- Changeable appetite
- Loss of appetite for months

craves alcohol

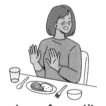
loss of appetite

RELATED REMEDIES
Mercury, Aurum, Nitric Acid, Fluoric Acid

139

Tubercular Miasm
Reaction

 The homeopathic remedy which is used to treat the Tubercular miasm is called TUBERCULINUM and it is a nosode made from the tissue of a Tuberculosis patient.

MENTAL PRESENTATION

- Easily bored
- Feels unfulfilled and restless
- Longs to find inner contentment
- Sensation seekers
- Desires change (yet not good with it)
- Needs freedom and to travel
- Grass is always greener - changes jobs, partners, house, courses
- Fear of animals especially dogs and cats
- Sensitive to music
- Violent temper
- Malicious
- Precocious, obstinate and disobedient children
- Hyperactive
- Headbanging children
- Depressed
- Curses and swears

needs freedom

desires change

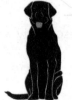

fear of dogs

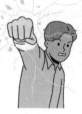

temper

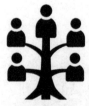

EVENT THAT CAUSED SYMPTOMS:

- Inherited miasm from ancestor
- History of tuberculosis

DREAMS:

- Mountains
- Animals

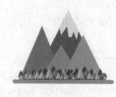

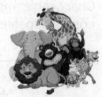

Tubercular Miasm
Reaction

KEYNOTES & PHYSICAL SYMPTOMS:
- Respiratory issues including pneumonia
- Skin issues such as eczema, ringworm
- Chronic, hard, short, dry, constant cough
- Sensation of suffocation
- Frequent colds and flu
- Perforated eardrum
- Reactive asthma (rather than mucus)
- Tonsillitis and enlarged tonsils
- Bedwetting
- Night sweats
- Allergies to animal hair and milk
- Consumption (yet looks healthy - red cheeks)
- Headbanging
- Teeth grinding
- Hypersexual
- Very long eyelashes and hairy back

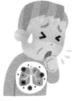

respiratory issues   **persistent cough**

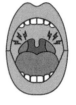 

tonsillitis   **allergies**

 damp   **mountain air**

Hindered by:
Change of weather
Cold, damp
On waking

Helped by:
Air in the mountains
Pine forests
Warm weather

FOOD:
- Craves smoked meat and bananas
- Loves cold milk yet allergies to dairy

craves smoked meat   **cold milk**

> **RELATED REMEDIES**
> Calc Phos, Drosera, Phosphorus,

141

Cancer Miasm
Suppression and boundaries

The homeopathic remedy which is used to treat the Cancer miasm is called CARCINOSIN and it is a nosode made from the discharge of breast cancer.

MENTAL PRESENTATION
- Passionate people who overgive
- Sensitive and sympathetic
- Poor boundaries
- Conformity
- Perfectionist
- People pleaser
- Fastidious - may have OCD
- Anticipatory anxiety
- Fear of disease and cancer
- Feels guilty
- Little anger (or may be suppressed)
- History of suppression
- Poor boundaries
- Lacks self-confidence
- Desires travel
- Loves music and dancing
- Loves thunderstorms

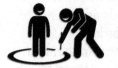
poor boundaries

people pleaser

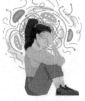
anxiety

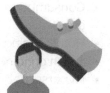
suppression

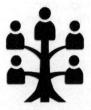
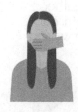

EVENT THAT CAUSED SYMPTOMS:
- Inherited miasm from ancestor
- History of cancer
- Sexual abuse or abusive relationship
- 'Glandular fever' or mononucleosis

DREAMS:
- Of being abused
- Of anger

Cancer Miasm
Suppression and boundaries

KEYNOTES & PHYSICAL SYMPTOMS:

- Warm blooded
- Immune system - overactive or underactive
- Multiple allergies
- Autoimmune issues
- Eczema
- Asthma
- Blood issues such as haemophilia, haemorrhages or pernicious anaemia
- Skin - eczema, moles, birthmarks, keloid scars, slow to heal wounds
- Infertility
- Suppression of previous illnesses
- Lack of childhood illnesses
- Chronic fatigue
- Insomnia and sleeplessness
- Tumours and polyps
- 'Never been well since' Glandular fever or mononucleosis

autoimmune issues

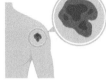

skin issues

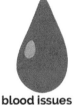

blood issues

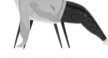

chronic fatigue

 full moon

 thunderstorms

Hindered by:
Warm room
Full or new moon

Helped by:
Open air
During thunderstorms
Seaside

FOOD:
- Craves butter and fat
- Desires chocolate

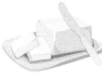

craves butter

craves chocolate

RELATED REMEDIES
Folliculinum, Natrum Mur, Staphisagria

A new Strep miasm?
Loss of self

Streptococcinum is a homeopathic nosode made from the bacteria Streptococcus pyrogenes.

MENTAL PRESENTATION

- OCD - which may have come on suddenly
- Obsessive
- Fear of wrongdoing
- Intrusive thoughts
- Perfectionism
- Separation anxiety
- Baby voice
- Regression
- Ritualistic behaviour
- Rage and tantrums
- Hates the sound of people eating and breathing
- Extreme sensitivity to noise
- Auditory hallucinations
- Dislikes praise
- Self critical
- Depressed
- Weeps on being given sympathy
- Highly strung
- Fears germs
- Homesickness

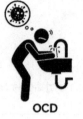

OCD

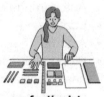

perfectionist

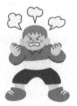

rage

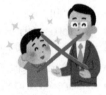

dislikes praise

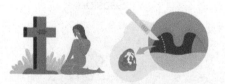

EVENT THAT CAUSED SYMPTOMS:

- History of strep related illnesses
- Tonsillectomy
- Suppressed grief in family or mother

There are over 50 different species of Streptococcus. It is possible to get homeopathic remedies made up of any of the species but the most commonly indicated is Streptoccous pyrogenes which is what the homeopathic remedy 'Streptococcinum' is made out of.

A new Strep miasm?
Loss of self

KEYNOTES & PHYSICAL SYMPTOMS:

- 'Never been well since' strep
- History of strep related illnesses
- Repeated tonsillitis, sore throats, quinsy, urinary tract infections or ear infections
- Chronic sore throats
- Thick mucus in back of throat
- Swollen tonsils, bad breath
- Susceptibility to colds
- Arthritis and joint pains
- Sinusitis
- Severe flu, pneumonia. bronchitis or pleurisy
- Tics, twitching, Tourette's, vocal stims
- Excessive thirst and urinating at night
- Chicken skin
- Stomach aches
- Headaches
- Scarlet fever

strep related illnesses

chronic sore throats

frequent colds

tics

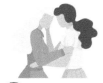

consolation

open air

Hindered by:
Consolation
Humid weather
Drafts
Wet weather
First movement

Helped by:
Continued movement
Open air

RELATED REMEDIES
Belladonna, Pyrogenium, Rhus Tox, Stramonium

Sarcodes

The following section provides an overview of the most commonly needed sarcodes including:

- Adrenalinum
- Cortisol
- Dopamine
- Folliculinum
- Glutamate
- Histaminum
- Oxytocin
- Pineal Gland
- Pituitary Gland
- Serotonin
- Testosterone
- Thymuline
- Thymus Gland
- Thyroidinum

Adrenalinum
Fight or flight

 Made from Adrenaline (or epinephrine) - a hormone and neurotransmitter produced by the adrenal glands that triggers the body's 'fight or flight' response.

MENTAL SYMPTOMS:

- Polar symptoms may present depending on whether there is too much or too little adrenaline
- Too little - timid, sad, tired, needs stimulants
- Too much - wants to run away, overexcitable, happy, hurried, needs physical activity to be able to sleep
- Anxiety and stress
- Pre-exam nerves
- Psychosis
- Poor concentration

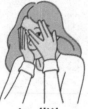 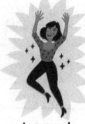

too little   **too much**

burnout   **migraines**

insomnia   **panic attacks**

KEYNOTES & PHYSICAL SYMPTOMS:

- Balances adrenaline levels
- Addicted to stimulants or exercise
- Panic attacks
- Palpitations
- Tachycardia
- High blood pressure
- Congestion of lungs including asthma
- Insomnia
- Migraines
- Burnout
- Constipation or diarrhoea

EVENT THAT CAUSED SYMPTOMS:

- Stress or threat
- Physical exertion
- Overenthusiasm

STRESS LEVEL

RELATED REMEDIES

Aconite, Coffea, Nitric Acid, Tuberculinum, Opium, Cortisol

Cortisol
Burnout

 Made from Cortisol - a steroid hormone produced by the adrenal glands that helps regulate metabolism, immune response, and stress, often referred to as the 'stress hormone.'

MENTAL SYMPTOMS:
- Perfectionists
- Those who go above and beyond
- Sense of duty
- Burnout
- Exhaustion
- Overthinking
- Mood swings
- Depression
- Extremely stressed

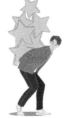

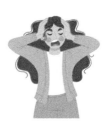

perfectionist   **stressed**

KEYNOTES & PHYSICAL SYMPTOMS:
- Balances cortisol
- Number 1 remedy for burnout
- Long-term stress
- Chronic fatigue syndrome
- Insomnia, fatigue and exhaustion
- Autoimmune issues
- History of hydrocortisone creams
- Craves carbohydrates
- May have high levels of Omega 6 fats
- History of exposure to radiation

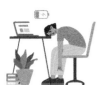

burnout   **chronic fatigue**

insomnia   **craves carbs**

EVENT THAT CAUSED SYMPTOMS:
- Stress
- Hydrocortisone creams

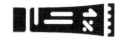

RELATED REMEDIES
Rhus Tox, Natrum Mur, Pulsatilla, Carcinosin, Nux Vomica, Psorinum, Adrenalinum

Dopamine
Addiction

Made from dopamine - a neurotransmitter in the brain that plays a key role in regulating mood, motivation, pleasure and reward, as well as various bodily functions like movement and attention.

MENTAL SYMPTOMS:
- Daredevils
- Addicted to thrills
- Craves excitement yet fears death
- Hyperactivity
- Highly stressed individuals
- Feels not good enough
- Concentration issues
- Fear of public speaking
- Blackouts during exams
- Hypochondria
- Depression

daredevils   stressed

KEYNOTES & PHYSICAL SYMPTOMS:
- Addiction in general - sugar, salt, alcohol, drugs, fat
- Screen addictions
- Conditions associated with low dopamine levels such as Parkinson's, Schizophrenia or ADHD
- Hyperactivity
- History of amniocentesis in pregnancy
- Jaundice after birth
- Restless legs
- Insomnia (the amazing homeopa Natasha Burns recommends a 30 or 200c before bedtime)

addictions   hyperactivity

diabetes   insomnia

EVENT THAT CAUSED SYMPTOMS:
- History of opiate use

RELATED REMEDIES
Aconite, Aurum, Belladonna, Carcinosin, Oxytocin

Folliculinum
'The hormonal Carcinosin'

A remedy made from the synthetic hormone oestrone, commonly used in contraceptive pills. Although this remedy is grouped with sarcodes, it is technically an isopathic remedy.

MENTAL SYMPTOMS:

- Often indicated when Carcinosin fails to act
- No sense of self or low self esteem
- Doormat - allow people to walk all over them
- Feels weight of peer pressure
- 'Rescuing' addiction - overwhelming need to help others at the cost of their own well-being
- Lacks self-control
- Bonding issues
- Child unable to separate from parent

no sense of self   **doormat**

pill side effects

eating disorders

PMS

menopause

KEYNOTES & PHYSICAL SYMPTOMS:

- 'Never been well since' the contraceptive pill
- Eating disorders
- Thrush with craving for sugar
- Symptoms appear, or are worse, from ovulation to menses
- Hormonal issues including ovarian cysts, PMS, migraine, menopause issues, menstrual problems, painful breasts, post-natal depression
- Migraines and congestive headaches

EVENT THAT CAUSED SYMPTOMS:

- Contraceptive pill
- Sexual, psychological or physical abuse

RELATED REMEDIES
Carcinosin, Lachesis, Sepia, Pulsatilla

Glutamate
The need to be in control

Made from Glutamate - an amino acid that acts as the primary excitatory neurotransmitter in the brain, playing a crucial role in learning, memory and overall brain function.

MENTAL SYMPTOMS:
- Needs to be in control of everything
- OCD
- Attention deficit disorder
- Trauma especially PTSD
- Burnout
- Cannot relax
- Hyperactivity
- Anxiety

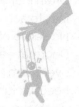

OCD **controlling**

exhaustion

sensory issues

insomnia **MSG side effects**

KEYNOTES & PHYSICAL SYMPTOMS:
- Burnout, exhaustion, fatigue
- Sensory processing issues
- PTSD
- High blood pressure
- Depression
- Insomnia
- Counteracts side effects of Monosodium Glutamate
- Migraines
- Conditions associated with high levels of Glutamate including Alzheimer's, ALS, epilepsy

EVENT THAT CAUSED SYMPTOMS:
- Monosodium Glutamate

RELATED REMEDIES
Ignatia, Natrum Mur, Merc, Plutonium, Syphylinum, Platina

Histaminum
Homeopathic anti-histamine

Other names: Histamine, Histamine hydrochloricum, Histaminum muriaticum
Histaminum is prepared from the chemical compound histamine.

MENTAL SYMPTOMS:
- Alienation and feeling like 'I don't belong'
- Nervous
- Rebellious
- Impatient
- Sensitive to slightest trifles
- Chameleon-like
- Restlessness

alienated

nervous

KEYNOTES & PHYSICAL SYMPTOMS:
- Leaky gut
- Mast cell activation syndrome
- Urticaria, allergic reactions, anaphylaxis
- Hayfever
- Eczema
- Dryness of mucus membranes
- Redness, burning and itching
- Unidentifiable stomach pain
- Burning in the nose, throat, ears
- Gluten intolerance
- Crohn's disease

urticaria

allergies

stomach pain

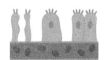
leaky gut

Hindered by:
Heat
Movement

Helped by:
Pressure
Fanning

heat

fanning

RELATED REMEDIES
Nux Vomica, Tarentula, Lachesis

Oxytocin
Bonding

 A remedy made from the synthetic form of oxytocin that is routinely given during childbirth. Although this remedy is grouped with sarcodes, technically it is an isopathic remedy.

MENTAL SYMPTOMS:
- Attachment issues
- Disconnection, separation and isolation
- Lack of maternal bonding
- Often indicated where no breastfeeding
- Communication issues including speech delays
- Lack of self love
- Issues sharing love
- Perfectionism
- Anxiety about making mistakes and feeling judged by others
- Fear of failure and losing control

lack of bonding   lack of self love

KEYNOTES & PHYSICAL SYMPTOMS:
- Endocrine and nervous system issues
- Out of balance oxytocin levels
- Infertility due to poor sperm function
- Breastfeeding issues including when stopping weaning
- Incontinence at night or during the day
- Poor muscle tone
- Pelvic instability
- Can be used to 'detox' side effects of artificial oxytocin

poor muscle tone   incontinence

balancing oxytocin   detoxing syntocin

EVENT THAT CAUSED SYMPTOMS:
- Syntocin during childbirth
- Lack of breastfeeding

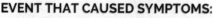

RELATED REMEDIES
Lac Maternum

Pineal Gland
Spiritual reconnection

 A sarcode made from the tissue of the pineal gland, an endocrine gland located in the center of the brain.

MENTAL SYMPTOMS:
- Disconnection from one's purpose
- Blocked intuition
- Restlessness and agitation without clear cause
- Obsessive thinking
- Easily distracted and overwhelmed
- Anxiety about the future and existential fears
- Emotional sensitivity
- Difficulty processing thoughts, feeling blocked or stuck
- Dependence on external validation
- Lack of motivation or direction
- Agitation after hallucinogenic or psychotropic drugs

 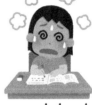

disconnection   **overwhelmed**

disorientation   **vertigo**

head pressure   **unresponsive chronic issues**

KEYNOTES & PHYSICAL SYMPTOMS:
- Endocrine and nervous system imbalance
- Sensory hypersensitivity
- Sleep disturbances and nightmares
- Disorientation and vertigo
- Head pressure and tinnitus
- Digestive issues linked to emotional stress
- Chronic conditions unresponsive to other remedies

EVENT THAT CAUSED SYMPTOMS:
- Hallucinogenic or psychotropic drug use

RELATED REMEDIES
Thymus Gland, Spectrum

Pituitary Gland
Growth

Other names: Pituitaria Glandula
A sarcode prepared from a macerated pituitary gland.

MENTAL SYMPTOMS:
- Mental weakness
- Poor concentration
- Nighttime anxiety
- Involuntary crying
- Fear of passing urine
- Fear of impotence
- Body dysmorphic disorder
- Obsessive

anxiety at night

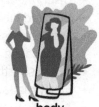

body dysmorphia

delayed growth

bedwetting

KEYNOTES & PHYSICAL SYMPTOMS:
- Delayed growth
- Delayed puberty and menses
- Undescended testicles
- High blood pressure
- Nighttime bedwetting
- Skin pigmentation issues - vitiligo or chloasma
- Painful periods
- Rectal spasms
- Alopecia
- Bleeding on the brain

hypertension   spasms

Hindered by:
Heat
Closed room
End of day

Helped by:
Fresh air
Open air

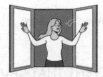

 heat   fresh air

RELATED REMEDIES
Baryta Carb, Ignatia, Thuja, Syphilinum

Serotonin
Depression

Made from serotonin - a neurotransmitter that helps regulate mood, sleep, appetite, and digestion, and is often associated with feelings of well-being and happiness.

MENTAL SYMPTOMS:

- Depression
- Anxiety
- Emotionally unbalanced
- Feels misunderstood
- Burnout
- Lacks self-confidence
- Hyperactivity
- Fear of speaking
- OCD
- Rituals and repetitiveness
- Difficulty focussing
- Argumentative

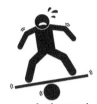

depression   **unbalanced**

KEYNOTES & PHYSICAL SYMPTOMS:

- 'Never been well since' SSRIs
- Very low or very high sex drive
- Painlessness, sensitivity to pain or chronic pain
- Fibromyalgia
- Insomnia
- Exhaustion
- Eating disorders
- Restlessness
- Sensory processing issues
- Mania
- Psychosis

exhaustion

fibromyalgia

insomnia

sexual dysfunction

EVENT THAT CAUSED SYMPTOMS:

- History of SSRIs
- Leaky gut (as 90% of serotonin is produced in the gut)

RELATED REMEDIES
Aurum, Dopamine, Natrum Mur

Testosterone
Balancing testosterone

Made from testosterone - a hormone primarily produced in the testes in males and in smaller amounts by females (in the ovaries and adrenal glands).

MENTAL SYMPTOMS:

- Thinks they know better than everyone else
- Competitive
- The innovator
- Easily angered
- Tough
- Melancholy - may cry
- Anti-social
- Dislikes getting older
- Depression
- Irritability

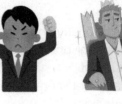

angry   arrogant

KEYNOTES & PHYSICAL SYMPTOMS:

- Loss of libido - helps increase sex drive
- Infertility
- Enlarged prostate
- Polycystic Ovarian Syndrome in women
- Hormonal acne
- Male pattern baldness
- Premature aging - wrinkles
- Loss of energy and fatigue
- Insomnia
- Osteoporosis

prostate issues   loss of libido

infertility   hormonal acne

EVENT THAT CAUSED SYMPTOMS:

- 'Manopause' - when men reach 40s/50s

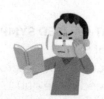

RELATED REMEDIES
Aurum, Platina, Sepia

Thymuline
Strengthen the body's defence

Made from the hormone thymulin, produced by the thymus gland, which supports T-cell development and helps maintain the body's internal balance and overall health.

MENTAL SYMPTOMS:

- Weak
- Lack of resilience
- Stressed
- This remedy is often prescribed as a therapeutic to help 'boost the immune system'

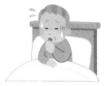

weak

stressed

boosts overall wellbeing

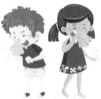

seasonal colds

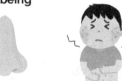

mucus

allergies

KEYNOTES & PHYSICAL SYMPTOMS:

- Enhances overall wellbeing
- Strengthens the body's defence during times of stress
- Useful for those who develop frequent seasonal colds and flu
- Slow recovery from illnesses
- Frequent illnesses
- Allergy symptoms
- Excess mucus
- Autoimmune issues

- Can use therapeutically in a low potency (9c or under) to support the body during times of stress or changes of season

RELATED REMEDIES
Silica, Tuberculinum

Thymus Gland
Unsuppresses

 Made from the thymus gland – a vital organ in the upper chest that plays a key role in maintaining the body's balance and overall health, especially during childhood.

MENTAL SYMPTOMS:

- This remedy opens one up to be able to process physical, mental and emotional past trauma
- Slow learners
- Obsessive over cleanliness
- Adults who have been cut off from ancestors - refugees
- Hopelessness
- Feels guilty
- Spacey

unsuppresses

hopelessness

circulation

trauma

brain injury

weight change

KEYNOTES & PHYSICAL SYMPTOMS:

- Affects circulation of body fluids, including lymph, water, blood and electrical energy
- Heals nervous system from trauma
- Long standing brain injury
- Sudden weight gain or loss
- Personality changes after medications, drugs or acute illnesses
- 'Never been well since' toxins, drugs or medications

EVENT THAT CAUSED SYMPTOMS:

- Medications
- Chicken pox or measles

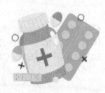

RELATED REMEDIES
Natrum Mur, Sepia, Aurum, Thuja

Thyroidinum
Thyroid issues

Other names: Thyroid gland extract, Thyroidea
A sarcode made from the thyroid gland of a sheep, ox or calf.

MENTAL SYMPTOMS:
- Developmental delays
- Feels they are being persecuted
- Quarrelsome with family
- Melancholy
- Irritable - 'goes into a rage over trifles'
- Difficulty concentrating
- Absent-minded
- Anxiety

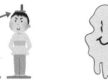

developmental delays   irritable

stunted growth   floppy babies

heart issues   goiter

KEYNOTES & PHYSICAL SYMPTOMS:
- Stunted growth
- Hypotonia - 'floppy' babies
- Endocrine issues
- Breast cysts
- Lack of breast milk
- Undescended testicles
- Uterine fibroids
- Heart issues - tachycardia, chest feels constricted
- Thyroid issues like goiter
- Nighttime bedwetting
- Eczema, psoriasis, brown swellings
- Alopecia

Hindered by:
Before menses
Stooping
Cold

Helped by:
After menses
Evening
Lying on stomach
Rest

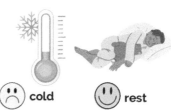

cold   rest

RELATED REMEDIES
Spongia, Calc Carb, Natrum Mur

Nosodes

The following section provides an overview of the most commonly
needed nosodes including:
- Babesia
- Bartonella
- Borrelia
- Candida Albicans
- Clostridium Difficile
- Influenzinum
- Lyssinum
- Mycoplasma
- Pertussinum
- Pneumococcinum
- Poly Fungi Plus
- Pyrogenium
- Staphylococcinum

Babesia
Oppression

 This nosode is made from the protozoa Babesia. It is commonly found to coincide alongside Borrelia and Bartonella.

MENTAL SYMPTOMS:
- Mood swings
- Dream like state
- Hallucinations
- Depression
- Anxiety
- Loss of concentration
- Agitated
- Confusion
- Despair

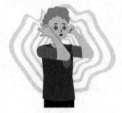

mood swings   **hallucinations**

KEYNOTES & PHYSICAL SYMPTOMS:
- Night sweats
- Gradual onset
- Fatigue
- Loss of appetite
- Joint pains
- Respiratory issues, including air hunger and shortness of breath
- Heart issues
- Chest pains and tightness
- Dark urine or jaundice caused by the breakdown of red blood cells
- Headache with a feeling of dizziness
- Angelica Lemke notes that 'for those who are immunosuppressed its manifestation can be severe cognitive impairment.'

night sweats

loss of appetite

slow onset

heart pains

EVENT THAT CAUSED SYMPTOMS:
- Tick bites

RELATED REMEDIES
China, Arsenicum, Natrum Mur

164

Bartonella
Darkness and fear

 This nosode is made out of the bacterium 'Bartonella' which is reputed to be transmitted by cat scratches and bites, also known as 'cat scratch disease'. It is commonly found to coincide alongside Borrelia.

MENTAL SYMPTOMS:

- Extremely dark - talk of death, zombies, suicide, devil
- Rage, screaming, hitting
- Psychosis as if an evil presence
- Intrusive thoughts
- Extreme fears
- Lack of empathy
- Confusion
- Mood swings at full moon

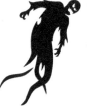

dark thoughts

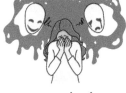

psychosis

psychosis

stretch mark rashes

KEYNOTES & PHYSICAL SYMPTOMS:

- Extreme states of mania or psychosis
- Tumours
- Skin rashes, especially those that look like stretch marks which disappear as suddenly as they appeared
- Flu-like symptoms and fevers
- Bone pain
- Urinary issues

urinary issues

bone pain

EVENT THAT CAUSED SYMPTOMS:

- Cat scratch or bite
- Fleas, ticks or mosquito bites

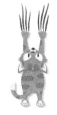

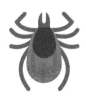

RELATED REMEDIES
Belladonna, Cina, Stramonium, Anacardium, Tarentula, Veratrum

165

Borrelia
The energetic imprint of Lyme Disease

 Other names: Borrelia burgdorferi, Lyme disease
A homeopathic nosode made from the spirochete bacterium Borrelia burgdorferi.

MENTAL SYMPTOMS:
- Cognitive decline
- Sensory processing issues and sensory sensitivity - to lights, sound, noise and touch
- OCD
- Tics
- Irritable and explosive
- Hyperactive and inattentive
- Phobias and fears
- Depression
- Anxiety, paranoia and suspicious - everyone is an enemy
- Brain fog
- Lack of motivation

OCD   sensory processing issues

heart issues   headaches

swollen glands   fatigue

KEYNOTES & PHYSICAL SYMPTOMS:
- Lyme disease
- 'Never been well since' a tick bite
- Fatigue and low energy
- POTS and/or dizziness
- Heart inflammation
- Migraines and headaches
- Floaters
- Fevers with no known cause
- Intolerance of hot or cold
- Night terrors
- Swollen glands
- Irritable bladder
- Dry non-productive cough
- Neurological disorders

EVENT THAT CAUSED SYMPTOMS:
- Tick bite

RELATED REMEDIES
Apis, Merc, Syphilinum, Ledum, Rhus Tox

Candida Albicans
Candida issues

Other name: Thrush fungus
A homeopathic nosode made from the fungus Candida Albicans.

MENTAL SYMPTOMS:
- Lack of boundaries
- Overburdened
- Melancholy
- Desires independence
- Doormat - allow people to walk all over them
- Giggling or silly behaviour

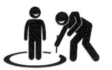

lack of boundaries

independent

KEYNOTES & PHYSICAL SYMPTOMS:
- Candidiasis, oral or vaginal thrush
- Bedwetting
- Teeth grinding
- Cradle cap
- Leucorrhoea
- Vaginitis
- Flatulence and gas
- Fluffy stools
- Bloated or rumbling abdomen
- Burning mouth, throat or genitals
- Pimples on bottom
- Toe walking
- Spinning
- Chemical sensitivity

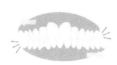

oral thrush   **teeth grinding**

flatulence

fluffy stools

EVENT THAT CAUSED SYMPTOMS:
- History of antibiotics

RELATED REMEDIES
Medhorrinum, Sepia, Saccharum

Clostridia Difficile
Gut dysbiosis linked to C. diff

 Other names: C. diff A homeopathic nosode made from the bacterium Clostridium difficile, which can cause diarrhoea symptoms, often after using antibiotics when the gut bacteria are out of balance.

MENTAL SYMPTOMS:

- Aggressive and threatening
- Instigates fights
- Desires isolation
- Self harm, including hitting and pinching
- Self hate
- Demanding
- Increased behavioural issues after antibiotics

aggressive   **self hate**

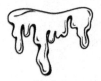

blood & mucus   **diarrhoea**

sensory seeking   **history of hospital stays**

KEYNOTES & PHYSICAL SYMPTOMS:

- Disrupted bowel movements after antibiotics
- Blood and mucus in stools
- Long term diarrhoea
- Sensory seeking
- Lemke notes there may be a 'history of prolonged hospital stays in child or someone in the family'

EVENT THAT CAUSED SYMPTOMS:

- Antibiotics

RELATED REMEDIES
Streptococcinum, Thuja, Anacardium

Influenzinum
All things 'flu' related

 A homeopathic nosode made from the secretions of individuals with 'influenza' symptoms.

MENTAL SYMPTOMS:
- Obsessions
- Delusions
- Anxious
- Brain fatigue
- Post-flu depressive neurosis

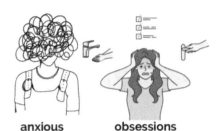

anxious   **obsessions**

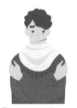 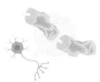

flu symptoms   nervous system issues

KEYNOTES & PHYSICAL SYMPTOMS:
- Typical flu symptoms - chills, headache, heavy eyes. aches and pains, weakness and fatigue, diarrhoea
- Nervous system symptoms and neurological issues following flu

EVENT THAT CAUSED SYMPTOMS:
- 'Never been well since' flu symptoms

- Use therapeutically for flu symptoms: 30c every 1–4 hours or as needed.
- Use homeoprophylactically as a preventative: 200c every 2–4 weeks

RELATED REMEDIES
Gelsemium, Oscillococcinum

Lyssinum
Never been well since a dog bite

Other names: Rabies nosode, Lyssin
A homeopathic nosode made from the saliva of a rabid dog.

MENTAL SYMPTOMS:
- Hypersensitive of all senses
- Extreme fear of water (hydrophobia)
- Wants water but can't drink
- Fears shiny objects, mirrors, church bells, driving, planes, insanity
- Extreme empathy
- Abusive, rude, bites and strikes
- Feels remorseful after rage
- Sensory issues - seams in socks irritate

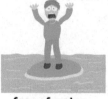

fear of water

sensory issues

KEYNOTES & PHYSICAL SYMPTOMS:
- 'Never been well since' a dog bite
- Weak back - feels as if it would spli
- Soreness in lower abdomen
- Prolapsed uterus
- Heat and burning in heart
- Difficulty breathing
- Spasms and gagging when trying t drink water
- Diarrhoea - symptoms are worse fr hearing or seeing running water
- Urine issues - desires to urinate wh seeing running water
- Yawns but not tired

weak back

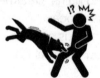

dog bites

EVENT THAT CAUSED SYMPTOMS:
- Dog bites
- Abuse

😞 water

🙂 rubbing

Hindered by:
Water - sight or sound of it running
Glistening objects

Helped by:
Bending backwards
Gentle rubbing

RELATED REMEDIES
Belladonna, Hyoscyamus, Stramonium, Lachesis

Mycoplasma
Respiratory issues

 A homeopathic nosode made from the bacterium Mycoplasma pneumoniae.

MENTAL SYMPTOMS:

- Depression
- Loneliness and isolation
- Tearful
- Puts up walls
- Withdrawn
- Anxiety
- Unsettled
- Feels worn down

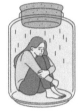 **depression**   **withdrawn**

KEYNOTES & PHYSICAL SYMPTOMS:

- Dry coughs
- Scratchy sore throat
- Copious perspiration with or without fever
- Fatigue
- Headache
- Chest feels sore
- Often indicated in those with a diagnosis of PANDAS/PANS or Lyme disease
- 'Never been well since' Mycoplasma

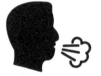 **dry coughs**   **sweaty**

 headache   **sore throat**

Mycoplasma is also known as 'walking pneumonia' due to its milder symptoms than typical 'pneumonia.' Use therapeutically for mycoplasma symptoms: 30c every 1–4 hours or as needed.

RELATED REMEDIES
Natrum Mur, Carcinosin, Pulsatilla

Pertussinum
Whooping cough ailments

 Other name: Pertussin, Whooping cough nosode
A homeopathic nosode made from the discharge of an individual with whooping cough ('pertussin').

MENTAL SYMPTOMS:
- Confusion
- Restlessness
- Tearful
- Feels guilty as if has done wrong
- Irritability
- Desperation

confusion

restless

KEYNOTES & PHYSICAL SYMPTOMS:
- Spasmodic coughing attacks
- Whooping cough therapeutic - can use alongside other indicated remedies
- Coughing fits that end with vomiting
- Tears with coughing
- Deep croupy cough

spasmodic cough

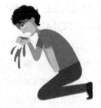
coughing that ends with vomiting

EVENT THAT CAUSED SYMPTOMS:
- 'Never been well since' whooping cough symptoms

- Use therapeutically for whooping cough symptoms: 30c every 2–4 hours or as needed
- Use homeoprophylactically as a preventative: 200c every 2–4 weeks

RELATED REMEDIES
Drosera, Ipecac

Pneumococcinum
Never been well since Pneumonia

 Other name: Pneumococcinum venenosum
A homeopathic nosode made from the bacterium
Pneumococcinum venenosum.

MENTAL SYMPTOMS:
- Depressed
- Weary of life
- Weak memory
- Does not want to go out of the home
- Fear of dying

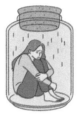

depressed   **wants to stay home**

KEYNOTES & PHYSICAL SYMPTOMS:
- Pneumonia
- Persistent headaches or altered mental state following pneumonia
- Stomach pains especially when hungry
- General respiratory issues
- Feels as if feather in throat
- Dry cough, worse in warm room
- Palpitations
- Headaches and left sinus pains
- Female - bearing down sensation
- Heavy legs

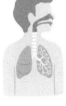

respiratory issues   **palpitations**

EVENT THAT CAUSED SYMPTOMS:
- 'Never been well since' pneumonia symptoms

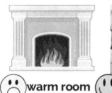
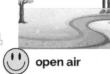

😟 **warm room**   🙂 **open air**

Hindered by:
Warm room
Humidity
Before menses
Inactivity

Helped by:
Open air, in the country
Short nap after meals
Hot foot bath

RELATED REMEDIES
Thuja, Medorrhinum

Poly Fungi Plus
To clear the energetic imprint of fungi

 A nosode made from a combination of mould, yeast and Clostridia Difficile created by the autism expert homeopath Wren Lloyd.

MENTAL SYMPTOMS:
- Uncontrollable laughing
- Giddiness
- Irritable
- Weeping
- Spaciness
- Tics
- OCD and intrusive thoughts
- Depression

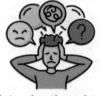

intrusive thoughts **giddiness**

KEYNOTES & PHYSICAL SYMPTOMS:
- Typically used to rebalance the body after mould exposure - this combination remedy also includes Clostridia Difficile to ensure gut remains balanced
- Recurrent chest symptoms
- Allergies and sneezing
- Picky eating
- Neurological inflammation
- Chronic sinusitis
- Loose stools
- Thrush or chronic candida
- Spitting
- Chewing clothes

allergies **sinusitis**

picky eating **loose stools**

EVENT THAT CAUSED SYMPTOMS:
- History of antibiotics
- Persistent mould exposure

Contains a mixture of: Candida albicans, Candida parapsilosis, Candida auris, Clostridium difficile, Alternaria alternata, Aspergillus niger, Aspergillus fumigatus, Fusarium spp., Serpula lacrymans, Mucor mucedo, Penicillium, Rhizopus nigricans, Sporobolomyces spp., Trichophyton rubrum, Ustilago spp., Cladosporium herbarum, house moulds, Stachybotrys chartarum, Torula spp., ringworm

Pyrogenium
Sepsis

Other name: Rotten meat
A homeopathic nosode made from the decomposition of chopped lean beef in water, allowed to stand in the sun for several weeks.

MENTAL SYMPTOMS:

- Confused
- Bed feels too hard
- Restless
- Delirium
- Semi-conscious with muttering
- Desires to be rocked
- Talks very fast
- Active mind

confused   **semi-conscious**

KEYNOTES & PHYSICAL SYMPTOMS:

- Sepsis
- Offensive discharges
- High fevers with delirium
- Food poisoning
- Abscesses
- Offensive menses, stools, vomiting
- Prolapsed uterus
- Retained placenta or fetus
- Septic symptoms after childbirth
- Threatened heart failure
- Septic cuts and bites

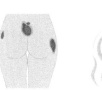

sepsis   **offensive discharges**

EVENT THAT CAUSED SYMPTOMS:

- Sepsis
- Miscarriage

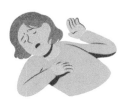

cold   **heat**

Hindered by:
Cold
Damp

Helped by:
Heat
Hot baths
Hot drinks
Pressure

RELATED REMEDIES
Arsenicum, Lachesis, Rhus Tox, Sulphur

Staphylococcinum
The energetic imprint of Staphylococcus

 A homeopathic nosode made from the bacterium Staphylococcus aureus.

MENTAL SYMPTOMS:
- Presents similar to Streptococcinum
- Self-hatred
- Victimised
- Overemotional
- Sexual shame

self-hatred

sexual shame

impetigo

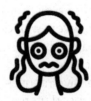
shakiness

KEYNOTES & PHYSICAL SYMPTOMS:
- Shakiness
- Restless sleep and dreams of dying
- Stomach cramps, gas and looseness
- Skin eruptions and itch
- Impetigo
- Fever and chills
- Hormonal acne
- Craves peanut butter

EVENT THAT CAUSED SYMPTOMS:
- A conflict where one feels soiled or attacked

- Use when there has 'never been well since' Staph
- Use therapeutically for 'Staph' symptoms: 30c every 4–6 hours or as needed

RELATED REMEDIES
Streptococcinum

The Bowel Nosodes

The following section provides an overview of the bowel nosodes which includes:

- Bacillus 7
- Colibacillinum/E-Coli/Mutabile
- Dysentry Co
- Gaertner
- Morgan Bach
- Morgan Gaertner
- Morgan Pure
- Proteus
- Sycotic Co

And the smaller remedies:

- Bacillus 10
- Faecalis

Bacillus No 7
Extreme fatigue and weakness

 Made from Bacillus asiaticus, Bacillus cloacae and Bacillus freundii. These are now known as Hafnia alvei, Enterobacter cloacae and Citrobacter freundii respectively.

MENTAL SYMPTOMS:
- Extreme weakness and fatigue - both mentally and physically
- Withdraws into self when there is perceived stress
- Tense and tired
- Lack of enjoyment of life
- Apathetic
- Just thinking of making any effort exhausts the individual
- Premature aging
- Severe tiredness
- Fixed ideas
- Premature senility
- Restless and unrefreshing sleep
- Takes hours to fall asleep then wakes at 2/3am

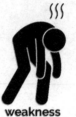

weakness

fatigue

apathetic

premature aging

EVENT THAT CAUSED SYMPTOMS:
- Severe illness
- Overindulgence

This bowel nosode was 'so named because it was the seventh group of non-lactose fermenting bacilli to be identified. Bacillus 10 was named for the same reason, but it must be remembered there is in fact no connections between the groups.' John Saxton

Bacillus No 7
Extreme fatigue and weakness

KEYNOTES & PHYSICAL SYMPTOMS:
- Fatigue, weakness, lethargy
- Chronic fatigue
- Sensitive to cold and draughts
- Poor muscle tone
- Premature dementia
- Senility
- Stiff joints which may crack, especially in neck
- Fibrous rheumatism of neck and back
- Faints easily when standing
- Low blood pressure
- Weak blood vessels resulting in burst veins
- Distended stomach and fullness after eating
- Backache
- Asthma worse at 2am
- Constipation
- Weak heart and slow pulse
- Thyroid issues
- Dull headaches
- Gout with debility
- Loss of sexual function

chronic fatigue

premature senility

poor muscle tone

stiff joints

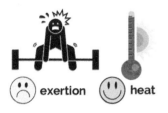

exertion   heat

Hindered by:	Helped by:
Middle of night	Rest
Stimulants	Heat
Eating	
Damp	
Exertion	

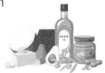

FOOD:
- Aversion to and aggravated by fats

aggravated by and aversion to fats

> **RELATED REMEDIES**
> Kali Carb, Rhus Tox

Colibacillinum, E.Coli, Mutabile
Sepsis

 E.Coli, Mutabile, Colibacillinum - 'symptoms are virtually indistinguishable' (Bickely) for these three nosodes and the key themes are septic states, infections and chronic UTIs.

MENTAL SYMPTOMS:

- Very timid
- Weariness
- Sadness
- Doubtful and hesitant
- Indecisive
- Gives up if doesn't succeed
- Passive
- Weak memory and confusion
- Struggles to find the right word
- Oppression, depressed and repressed
- Anxiety and phobias of crowds, open spaces
- Delusion he is poor
- Dreams of being stabbed
- Psychosis
- Out of touch with reality

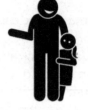
timid

weak memory

weariness

oppressed

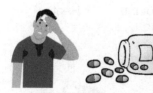

EVENT THAT CAUSED SYMPTOMS:

- Loss of fluids
- Overuse of antibiotics

This is one of the number one remedies for chronic UTIs and cystitis. Just a few doses of 200c potency has been known to work wonders for 'stuck' cases of chronic cystitis.

Colibacillinum, E.Coli, Mutabile
Sepsis

KEYNOTES & PHYSICAL SYMPTOMS:
- Septic states
- Alternating symptoms
- Very chilly
- Dementia
- Psychosis
- Food poisoning
- Rumbling stomach and flatulence
- Dehydrated babies with diarrhoea
- Loose spluttering stools
- Nausea and vomiting
- Bladder and kidney issues
- Chronic cystitis
- Frequent, urgent urination with little urine and urging to urinate just after urinating
- Painful urination with burning at the end
- Blood in the urine
- Feverishness with weakness
- Coated white tongue

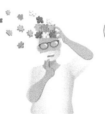

dementia　　**psychosis**

 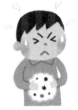

urine issues　**food poisoning**

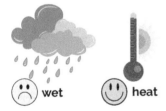

wet　**heat**

Hindered by:
Wet cold
Humidity
After rest
At seaside

Helped by:
Heat

FOOD:
- Aggravated by eggs, dairy and fish

fish aggravates　**egg aggravates**

> **RELATED REMEDIES**
> Arsenicum, China, Pyrogen, Sepia

Dysentry Co
Anxiety

FULL NAME: Dysentry Bacillus
Other name: Shigella dysenteria
Prepared from Bacillus dysenteriae which can be found in the intestinal region of the body.

MENTAL SYMPTOMS:

- Extremely fearful, especially of anything beyond their control
- Nervousness
- Anxiety, especially surrounding new events or people
- Avoidant behaviour, not just of challenges, but anything new
- Fear of failure
- Perfectionist
- Easily flustered
- Blushes with embarrassment
- Brain fatigue
- Shy and lacks self-confidence
- Restlessness and inability to relax
- Fear of being alone yet aggravated by consolation
- Very sensitive and can overreact especially to criticism
- Claustrophobic
- Obsessive compulsive disorder

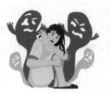
fearful

nervous

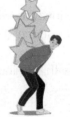
perfectionist

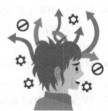
restless

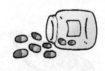

EVENT THAT CAUSED SYMPTOMS:
- Excess use of antibiotics

Whereas Proteus' tension usually comes from external factors, Dysentry Co's is internally self generated due to over-worry.

Dysentry Co
Anxiety

KEYNOTES & PHYSICAL SYMPTOMS:
- Anticipatory and performance anxiety
- Nervous tension - worry that sits in the stomach
- Digestive system issues - bloating, diarrhoea, colitis, chronic indigestion, heartburn
- Tension in stomach and heart
- Heart issues - palpitations and tachycardia
- Air hunger
- Sensitive to pain
- Insomnia
- Tics and twitches
- Frequent urination
- Migraines of nervous origin
- Chilly yet overheats and perspires easily

heart issues

tics

performance anxiety

digestive system issues

:(**3-6am**   :) **open air**

Hindered by:
3am-6am
Crowds
Consolation
Eating
Excitement

Helped by:
Open air
Warmth
Urination

FOOD:
- Desires cold drinks, sweets and fats which often aggravate

craves sweets & cold drinks yet aggravates

RELATED REMEDIES
Arg Nit, Arsenicum, Carcinosin, Lycopodium

Gaertner
Malabsorption and failure to thrive

FULL NAME: Gaertner Bacillus
Other names: Salmonella enteritidis
Prepared from Bacillus Salmonella enteritidis which can be found in the intestinal region of the body.

MENTAL SYMPTOMS:
- Nervous activity
- Restless
- Hyperactive
- Overactive mind
- Hypersensitive to both emotional and physical stimuli
- Hold onto emotional traumas
- Lacks confidence
- Pessimistic
- Anxious
- Precocious children
- Intelligent
- Sense of unease
- Likes routine
- Difficulty concentrating
- Unreliable yet wants to please
- Fear of heights
- Fear of being alone
- Night terrors
- Sleepwalking

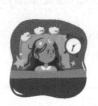
restless

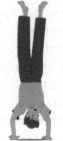
hyperactive

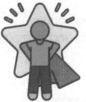
precocious children

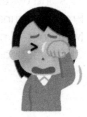
hypersensitive

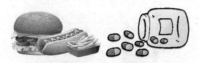

EVENT THAT CAUSED SYMPTOMS:
- Overuse of antibiotics
- Processed food

Gaertner is a bowel nosode derived from the specific bacterial strain, Salmonella enteritidis. This is a different remedy from Morgan Gaertner which combines elements of both Morgan Pure and aspects attributed to the Gaertner group!

Gaertner
Malabsorption and failure to thrive

KEYNOTES & PHYSICAL SYMPTOMS:
- Use therapeutically for 'never been well since' non-penicillin based antibiotics
- Malabsorption and failure to thrive
- Nutritional deficiencies in children
- Thin and undernourished
- Coeliac disease
- Digestive issues incl IBS, Crohn's
- Allergies especially to dairy
- Ketosis
- Nail biting
- Vomiting or pain in stomach
- Acid attacks
- Loose floating stools
- Blood and mucus in stool
- Recurrent or persistent worms especially threadworms
- Repeated ear infections especially with discharges
- For children who get ear discharge when teething

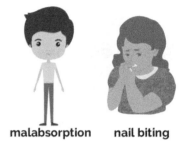

malabsorption   nail biting

antibiotic   recurrent
poisoning   threadworms

storms

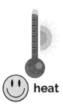
heat

Hindered by:
Animal fats
Cold and
stormy weather

Helped by:
Company
Heat

FOOD:
- Limited diet
- Desires oatmeal, cheese, eggs, milk, sugar
- Averse to bread, butter, meat, fish

desires oatmeal   averse to butter

RELATED REMEDIES
Silica, Carcinosin, Phosphorus

Morgan Bach
Congestion

FULL NAME: Morgan Bach
Prepared from Morgan Pure and the compound
Morgan Gaertner to make the new compound
Morgan Bach.

MENTAL SYMPTOMS:

- Introspective
- Nervous tension
- Restlessness
- Desires being active
- Generalised anxiety
- Health anxiety
- Depressed
- May desire to commit
  suicide by jumping
- Pessimistic
- Irritable
- Weeping and tearful
- Fear of crowds and
  agoraphobia
- Claustrophobia
- Dislikes being alone
- Insomnia or restless sleep
- Craves sleep after a meal

introspective

fear of crowds

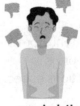
pessimistic

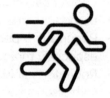
active

EVENT THAT CAUSED SYMPTOMS:

- Excess use of antibiotics
- Pneumonia

There is considerable overlap between Morgan Pure and Morgan
Gaertner - Morgan Bach is a compound of the two of them. Many
homeopaths use Morgan Bach, unless Morgan Pure or Morgan
Gaertner screams out as a better more specific fit.

Morgan Bach
Congestion

KEYNOTES & PHYSICAL SYMPTOMS:
- General congestion and sluggishness
- Skin issues such as eczema, boils, fissures, acne, herpes, impetigo, dermatitis
- Severe itching and raw skin that discharges
- Dry, cracked skin especially on the face
- Congestive headaches with flushing
- Overproduction of mucus which may present as heartburn, coated tongue or reflux
- Nasal or respiratory congestion, including recurrent bronchitis, asthma
- Haemorrhoids, piles, Bartholinitis, varicose veins
- Meniere's disease
- Constipation
- Gallstones
- Joint issues, including knees, wrists and fingers
- Menopausal - hot flushes, migraines
- Headaches worse for thunder

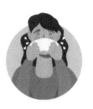

congestion   **skin issues**

bronchitis   **constipation**

 heat

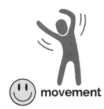 movement

Hindered by: **Helped by:**
Heat of the bed Movement
Night
Washing
Wool

FOOD:
- Desires fats, sweets, eggs, butter
- Fats and eggs aggravate

craves fats & eggs but aggravates

RELATED REMEDIES
Sulphur, Psorinum, Calc Carb, Lycopodium

Morgan Gaertner
Biliousness

> **FULL NAME: Morgan Gaertner**
> Prepared from Morgan Pure and Gaertner which can be found in the intestinal region of the body, to make the compound Morgan Gaertner.

MENTAL SYMPTOMS:
- Impatient
- Restless
- Tense
- Very critical and blunt
- Moans and complains
- Jealous
- Self-centered and self-pitying - feels deserves more than what life has given
- Irritable and short tempered
- Manic depression
- Fearful at night - may scream out in sleep
- Limited trust in health professionals
- Anticipatory anxiety
- Apprehensive
- Excitable in company
- Strong reactions
- Claustrophobic

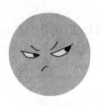

jealous

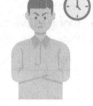

impatient

self-pitying

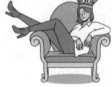

selfish

EVENT THAT CAUSED SYMPTOMS:
- Excess use of antibiotics
- Antacids

There is considerable overlap between Morgan Pure and Morgan Gaertner - Morgan Bach is a compound of the two of them. Many homeopaths use Morgan Bach, unless Morgan Pure or Morgan Gaertner screams out as a better more specific fit.

Morgan Gaertner
Biliousness

KEYNOTES & PHYSICAL SYMPTOMS:
- Biliousness
- Gallstones
- Stomach ulcers
- Offensive, brown and corrosive discharges
- One-sided complaints
- Waterbrash and belching
- Reflux/indigestion
- Bitter taste in the mouth
- Constipation with hard dry stools
- Recurrent tonsillitis
- Nail biting
- Headaches and migraines
- Nasal catarrh
- Nosebleeds caused by hard mucus
- Headaches with flushes of heat
- Rheumatism and arthritis
- Kidney pains
- Strong odour to urine
- Palpitations that wake from sleep
- Hair loss

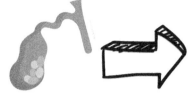

biliousness   right sided

reflux   constipation

 4-8pm   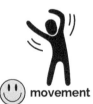 movement

Hindered by:
Excitement
Company
4-8pm
Eating
Before menses

Helped by:
Movement
Passing wind

FOOD:
- Craves sweets, salt and spicy food
- Averse to butter and eggs
- Feels full after eating little

craves sweets   averse butter

RELATED REMEDIES
Lycopodium. Chelidonium, Natrum Mur,
Nux Vomica, Pulsatilla, Silica

189

Morgan Pure
Congestion and issues from Penicillin

FULL NAME: Morgan Pure
Prepared from the gut bacterium Morganella morganii, a member of the Enterobacteriaceae family, commonly found in the intestinal tract.

MENTAL SYMPTOMS:

- Mental congestion
- Introspective
- Unstable
- Easily pushed into gloom
- Can't easily express feelings
- Inefficient communication
- Dwells on disagreeable thoughts
- Deeply anxious
- Health anxiety
- Fears of disease and overly worried about diet
- Overwhelmed by decisions and indecisive
- Fear of crowds
- Agoraphobia or claustrophobia
- Aimlessly active
- Worse when alone but averse to company

introspective

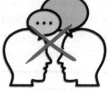
poor communication

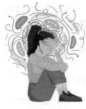
anxious

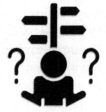
indecisive

EVENT THAT CAUSED SYMPTOMS:
- Excess use of Penicillin-based antibiotics
- Pneumonia

There is considerable overlap between Morgan Pure and Morgan Gaertner - Morgan Bach is a compound of the two of them. Many homeopaths use Morgan Bach, unless Morgan Pure or Morgan Gaertner screams out as a better more specific fit.

Morgan Pure
Congestion and issues from Penicillin

KEYNOTES & PHYSICAL SYMPTOMS:
- Use therapeutically for 'never been well since' Penicillin-based antibiotics
- Congestion and sluggishness
- Chronic skin issues
- Major remedy for eczema in children
- Moist skin
- Chronic liver issues, jaundice and gallstones
- Bronchitis and pneumonia, especially in the spring
- Kidney stones
- Strokes and thrombosis
- Periodic migraines, normally weekly
- Headaches which are worse from travelling
- Asthmatic tendency

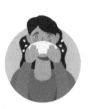

congestion

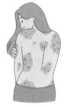

skin issues

eczema in babies

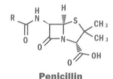

Penicillin

'never been well since' Penicillin

storms

eating

Hindered by:
Storms
Night
Morning
Humidity
Washing
Heat

Helped by:
Eating
Movement

FOOD:
- Desires fats, sweets, eggs, butter
- Fats and eggs aggravate

craves fats & eggs but aggravates

> **RELATED REMEDIES**
> Sulphur, Psorinum, Medorrhinum

Proteus
Suddenness

 FULL NAME: Proteus Bacillus
Prepared from a culture of a bacterium of the Proteus genus which is found in the intestinal region of the body.

MENTAL SYMPTOMS:
- 'Brainstorm' or temper tantrums
- Anthony Bickley states 'Nux Vomica on a bad day could be 'a mild Proteus tantrum'
- Hysteria
- Overwhelmed by stress
- Stress builds up slowly to be released violently
- Anxiety, irritability and depression
- Can lose control easily
- Family around them 'walks on eggshells'
- Loves routine
- Fixed ideas and stubborn
- Wants to be in control
- Disconnected, self-absorbed or detached
- Anger from contradiction
- Sensitive to criticism
- Aversion to company
- Lacks self-confidence

brainstorm

stressed

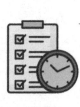
needs routine

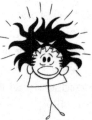
hysteria

EVENT THAT CAUSED SYMPTOMS:
- Long periods of external stressors
- Grief
- Bereavement

DREAMS:
- Violent dreams
- Death, destruction and murder
- Of people from the past

Proteus
Suddenness

KEYNOTES & PHYSICAL SYMPTOMS:
- Suddenness of mental or physical symptoms
- Slow recovery
- Nervous system issues
- Stress, anxiety and tension
- Cramps and spasms
- Convulsions and epilepsy
- Skin issues especially herpes or boils that are slow to mature
- Migraines with flashing lights
- Frontal headaches and pressing pains
- Heartburn
- Diarrhoea from emotional upset
- Food allergies
- Raynaud's syndrome
- Photophobia
- UTIs with cloudy urine or white sediment

suddenness   **spasms**

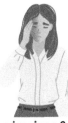 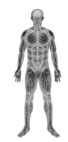

migraines & headaches   **nervous system issues**

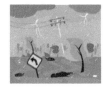 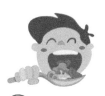

Hindered by:
Storms
Extremes of temperature

Helped by:
Resting
Being in mountains
Stretching
Eating

☹ storms   ☺ eating

FOOD:
- Aversion to eggs, dairy, raw food, chocolate, beef, pork, green vegetables
- Craves sweets and fats

aversion to eggs   **craves sweets**

RELATED REMEDIES
Natrum Mur, Aurum, Ignatia, Nux Vomica

Sycotic Co
Irritation

> **FULL NAME: Sycotic Co. Bacillus. Other names: Bacillus streptococcus faecalis**
> Made from Streptococcus faecalis found in the intestines.

MENTAL SYMPTOMS:

- Irritable
- Nervous, tense and easily upset
- Ailments from anticipation
- Exhaustion from worrying
- Restless
- Fussy - things must be just so
- Shy and sensitive, yet may desire the limelight
- Loses temper easily, especially when feeling resentful
- Hides fears and weaknesses
- Sibling rivalry
- Fears animals and dogs
- Fears being left alone
- Fears the dark
- Bites nails
- Hypochondriac

irritable

fussy

shy

fears dogs

EVENT THAT CAUSED SYMPTOMS:

- Overuse of antibiotics
- Suppression of acute illnesses

Sycotic Co is often compared to Thuja because both remedies address the sycotic miasm, dealing with conditions like warts, overgrowths or chronic imbalances, where there is a tendency towards 'excess' and also suppressed ailments.

Sycotic Co
Irritation

KEYNOTES & PHYSICAL SYMPTOMS:
- Overproduction issues such as warts, verruca, acne, polyps, cysts
- Overproduction of mucus - glue ear, sinusitis, ear wax
- Asthma especially worse for damp or between 2-3am
- Chronic candida
- Lumbo-sacral back pain
- Painful soles of feet
- Skin issues - ringworm, molluscum contagion, athlete's foot, dermatitis
- Respiratory issues such as pneumonia, bronchitis, pleurisy
- 'Strep B infections'
- Genital herpes
- Foul loose stools
- Fibrositis
- Chronic and recurring cystitis
- Long lasting nosebleeds with no known origin
- Alopecia
- Sweating at night

asthma   **excess mucus**

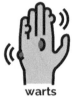 

warts   **candida**

  damp   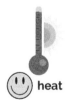 **heat**

Hindered by:	Helped by:
Cold	Heat
Damp	Seaside
First motion	
Night	

FOOD:
- Desire vinegar
- Egg aggravates
- Picky eater

desire vinegar   **egg aggravates**

> **RELATED REMEDIES**
> Thuja, Nitric Acid, Medorrhinum

195

Bacillus No 10
Poisonings and trauma

 Bacillus 10 is considered to be a more minor bowel nosode. There is no information available about the identity of the bacterium from which this nosode was prepared.

MENTAL SYMPTOMS:

- Anxious
- Overactive mind
- Irritable
- Depressed
- Fastidious and obsessive
- Sensitivity
- Heavy personality

irritable   **fastidious**

KEYNOTES & PHYSICAL SYMPTOMS:

- Ailments from poisoning
- Gallbladder pain
- Sluggish bowels
- Morning cough
- Asthma
- Tender coccyx
- Dry raw genitals
- Warts on hands
- Ringworm
- Anorexia from self-loathing
- Averse to breakfast

tender coccyx   **ailments from poisonings**

FOOD:

- Aversion to eggs, bread, tomatoes, tea
- Craves sweets, chocolate, fried fish

craves sweets   **averse eggs**

EVENT THAT CAUSED SYMPTOMS:

- Salmonella poisoning
- Internal trauma including rape and poisoning

RELATED REMEDIES
Calc Fluor

Faecalis
Sluggishness

 Faecalis is considered to be a more minor bowel nosode. It is made from a preparation of the bacterium Enterococcus faecalis, found in the human intestinal tract and is part of the normal gut flora

MENTAL SYMPTOMS:
- Sluggishness
- Lack of flexibility in thinking
- Unreceptive to new ideas or change
- Irritable
- Suppressed anger

fixed ideas   **irritable**

KEYNOTES & PHYSICAL SYMPTOMS:
- Sluggish
- Under-functioning vital force, which may present as a lack of reaction
- Slow digestion
- Haemorrhoids
- Liver issues especially after consuming fats
- Excess acid
- Chilly
- Unrefreshing sleep

sluggish   **lack of reaction**

FOOD:
- Aggravated by sweets, fats and sugars

aggravated by sweets   **aggravated by fats**

RELATED REMEDIES

Sepia

Isopathic Remedies

The following section provides a brief snapshot into isopathic remedies, illustrated with Chlorum Aqua, a combination remedy 'Poly Contraceptives' (poly means 'many') and an overview of some of the other most commonly-needed isopathic remedies.

It is important to note that it is possible to make a remedy out of almost any toxin, medication or drug.

Chlorum Aqua
For Chlorine exposure

 Made from Chlorine water.

MENTAL SYMPTOMS:
- Irritability
- Loss of memory
- Anger
- Quiet alternating with restlessness

irritability   **anger**

KEYNOTES & PHYSICAL SYMPTOMS:
- Typically used following exposure to chlorinated water
- Burning mucous membranes
- Watery eyes
- Excessive tears
- Irritated eyes and throat
- Dry, itchy skin
- Dry mouth
- Respiratory tightness
- Sensation of suffocation
- Nausea after drinking water
- Stinging skin eruptions
- Cough from inhaling vapours
- Relieved in fresh air
- Aggravated by humidity

running tears   **irritated eyes**

sense of suffocation   **cough**

EVENT THAT CAUSED SYMPTOMS:
- Chlorinated swimming pools

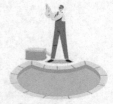

RELATED REMEDIES
Chlorum - Chlorum addresses symptoms from chlorine gas exposure, while Chlorum Aqua focuses on symptoms from exposure to chlorinated water.

Poly Contraceptives
To clear the energetic imprint of contraceptives

 Made from a combination of hormonal contraceptive pills.

MENTAL SYMPTOMS:

- Mood swings
- Low libido
- Can be one of two extremes - a 'Boss babe' or very subservient
- Loss of feminity
- Depression

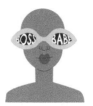

boss babes　　**depression**

PCOS　　　**infertility**

skin issues　　**PMS**

KEYNOTES & PHYSICAL SYMPTOMS:

- Typically used to rebalance the body after stopping the contraceptive pill
- Almost any hormonal issue
- Endometriosis
- Polycystic Ovary Syndrome
- Infertility
- Delayed or irregular menses
- Pre-menstrual tension
- Migraines
- Painful breasts
- Skin pigmentation

EVENT THAT CAUSED SYMPTOMS:

- Contraceptive pill

RELATED REMEDIES
Carcinosin, Lachesis, Sepia, Pulsatilla, Phytolacca, Folliculinum

Other Common Toxins
that are available as isopathic remedies

 POLY MRNA - helps clear side effects of MRNA products. This is the most important layer to treat and should be 'detoxed' first.

 POLY STEROIDS - helps clear side effects of steroids. After MRNA products, this is the most important layer to clear (along with poly contraceptives).

 POLY ANTIBIOTICS - contains a mixture of common antibiotics. Helps clear side effects of antibiotics. Symptoms may include leaky gut, skin issues, anxiety.

 ULTRASOUND - helps clear side effects of ultrasounds. Ultrasounds may reduce brain development and levels of dopamine. .

 POLY ENVIRONMENTAL RADIATION - helps clears side effects of radiation and includes a combination of remedies made from wifi, 3G, 4G, 5G, cosmic radiation.

 POLY METALS - while ideally the offending metal can be detoxed individually, this combination remedy contains a mixture of common heavy metals.

This is a tiny snapshot of the isopathic remedies that are available. It is pretty much possible to make an isopathic remedy out of any toxin, medication or drug.

These remedies should only be prescribed by a homeopath experienced in homeopathic detox.

202

Bibliography and references

Bibliography and references

- Allen, H.C. (1980). Keynotes. B. Jain Publishers.
- Assilem, M. (2009). Gifts of the Mother. Matridonal Remedies of the Humanum Family. Helios Pharmacy.
- Ang, E. S., Jr., Gluncic, V., Duque, A., Schafer, M. E., & Rakic, P. (2006). Prenatal exposure to ultrasound waves impacts neuronal migration in mice. Proceedings of the National Academy of Sciences, 103(34), 12903-12910.
- Austin, V. (2024). The Living Language of Water. Veda Austin Publishing.
- Bailey, P. (1995). Lac Remedies in Practice. Winter Press.
- Bickley, A. (2006). Bowel Nosodes: A Practice Handbook. B. Jain Publishers.
- Bracho, G., Varela, E., Fernández, R., Ordaz, B., Marzoa, N., Menéndez, J., Garcia, L., Gilling, E., Leyva, R., Rufín, R., de la Torre, R., Solis, R. L., Batista, N., Borrero, R., & Campa, C. (2010). Large-scale application of highly-diluted bacteria for Leptospirosis epidemic control. Homeopathy, 99(3), 156-166.
- Canniff, J., Fairley, C., Timms, P., & Hocking, J. (2011). Protective effect of chickenpox against cancers. Journal of Infection, 63(4), 284-292.
- Chappell, P. (2003). Emotional Healing with Homeopathy: Healing the Effects of Trauma. Winter Press.
- Clarke, J.H. (1902). The Cure and Prevention of Scarlet Fever.
- Dias, B. G., & Ressler, K. J. (2013). Parental olfactory experience influences behavior and neural structure in subsequent generations. Nature Neuroscience, 17(1), 89-96. DOI: 10.1038/nn.3594
- Emoto, M. (2004). The Hidden Messages in Water. Atria Books.
- Griffith, C. (2006). The New Materia Medica: Key Remedies for the Future of Homeopathy. Watkins Publishing
- Griffith, C. (2011). The New Materia Medica: Key Remedies for the Future of Homeopathy. Volume 2. Watkins Publishing
- Griffith, C. (2023). The New Materia Medica: Key Remedies for the Future of Homeopathy. Volume 3. Watkins Publishing
- Hahnemann, S. (1996). The Organon of the Medical Art (6th ed.). Translated by Wenda Brewster O'Reilly. Birdcage Books
- Jansen, T. (2016). Fighting Fire with Fire. Emryss Publishers.
- Jansen, T. (2021). Human Chemistry: Integrated Therapy from a Homeopathic Perspective. Emryss Publishers.
- Julian, O.A. (1979). Materia Medica of New Homeopathic Remedies. B. Jain Publishers.
- Kantor, J. M. (2022). Sane Asylums: The Success of Homeopathy before Psychiatry Lost Its Mind. Healing Arts Press.
- Kaznacheev, V. P., Mikhailova, L. P., & Kartashov, N. B. (1980). Distant intercellular electromagnetic interaction between two tissue cultures. Bulletin of Experimental Biology and Medicine, 89(3), 345–348.
- Lemke, A. (2020). Healing Complex Children with Homeopathy. Independent publication.

Bibliography and references

- Lester, D., & Parker, D. (2019). What Really Makes You Ill?: Why Everything You Thought You Knew About Disease Is Wrong. What Really Makes You Ill.
- Linde, K., Clausius, N., Ramirez, G., Melchart, D., Eitel, F., Hedges, L. V., & Jonas, W. B. (1997). Are the clinical effects of homoeopathy placebo effects? A meta-analysis of placebo-controlled trials. The Lancet, 350(9081), 834-843.
- McKusick, E. (2014). Tuning the Human Biofield: Healing with Vibrational Sound Therapy. Healing Arts Press.
- McKusick, E. D. (2021). Electric Body, Electric Health: Using the Electromagnetism Within (and Around) You to Rewire, Recharge, and Raise Your Voltage. St. Martin's Essentials.
- Morrison, R. (1993). Desktop Guide to Keynotes and Confirmatory Symptoms. Hahnemann Clinic Publishing.
- Murphy, R. (2006). Nature's Materia Medica (3rd ed.). Lotus Health Institute.
- Peppler, A. (2008). The Psychological Significance of Homeopathic Remedies. Narayana Publishers.
- Peppler, A. (2002). Creative Homeopathy: Volume 1. Institute of Creative Homeopathy.
- Phatak, S.R. (2002). Phatak's Materia Medica of Homoeopathic Medicines. B. Jain Publishers.
- Ronne, T. (1985). Measles virus infection without rash in childhood is related to a decreased risk of adult onset diseases. Lancet, 326(8440), 1-5.
- Rozencwajg, J. (2012). The Fibonacci Potency Series: The Renewed Science of Homeopathy. Emryss Publishers.
- Roytas, D. (2024). Can You Catch a Cold?: Exploring the Science and Myths of Colds and Flu. Daniel Roytas Publishing.
- Sankaran, R. (1991). The Spirit of Homeopathy. Homeopathic Medical Publishers.
- Saxton, J. (2013). Bowel Nosodes in Homeopathic Practice. Saltire Books.
- Silverberg, J. I., Silverberg, N. B., Lee-Wong, M., & Silverberg, M. S. (2012). Chickenpox infection and reduced risk of some cancers. Journal of Pediatrics, 161(6), 1109-1115.
- Smits, T. (2010). Inspiring Homeopathy: Treatment of Universal Layers. Emryss Publishers.
- Tabrett, D. (2017). Burnett Rediscovered: Clinical Strategies of the Great Homeopath for Modern Practice – Line of Action of Remedies – Organ Remedies – Pathological Similimum – Vaccinosis. Emryss Publishers..
- Vermeulen, F. (2018). Monera - Kingdom Bacteria and Viruses: Spectrum Materia Medica Volume 1. Narayana Publishers.
- Watson, I. (2004). A Guide to the Methodologies of Homeopathy. Cutting Edge Publications.
- Watson, I. (2009). The Homeopathic Miasms: A Modern View. Cutting Edge Publications.
- West, R. R. (1996). Mumps and ovarian cancer: Modern interpretation of a historic association. Epidemiology, 7(4), 440-442.

Appendix
How to dose for acute issues

Dosing for Acute Illnesses - Guidelines

> Dosing homeopathic remedies can take some getting used to because, unlike allopathic Western medicine, there are no set regimes or protocols. It is crucial to listen to the body and to see how it responds to the remedy. Depending on the individual and the nature of the symptoms, sometimes just one dose is all that is needed, yet at other times the remedy may need repeating frequently such as every 15 minutes. Below are some general dosing guidelines for intense acute illnesses.

DOSING GUIDELINES:

- Remember to ALWAYS LISTEN TO THE BODY
- For intense acute symptoms, give every 15-60 minutes and reduce as the symptoms improve
- For slower paced acute symptoms, give every 1-4 hours and reduce as the symptoms improve
- STOP when definite improvement is maintained
- If you have given 3-4 doses and there is NO improvement, then try a different remedy
- If symptoms do return, resume giving the remedy

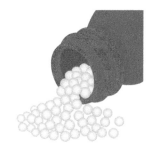

POTENCY:

- Ideally use 30c - it is a brilliant universal potency
- 12c can be used if 30c is not available, but it may need repeating more often
- 200c can be suitable for high intensity acute situations, especially where there are strong mental symptoms, such as childbirth

 ALWAYS STOP TAKING THE REMEDIES ONCE YOU FEEL BETTER

How to Dose for Acutes

THE LAW OF THE MINIMUM DOSE - Less is more!
Generally, give one pill and WAIT to see results and assess the effects of the remedy. If you feel much better after a dose, stop taking the remedy until the first sign that your symptoms have returned. You can keep repeating the remedy until a definite improvement is maintained.

When do I repeat the remedy?
Repeat the remedy when improvement stalls or the same symptoms return. In intense acute situations, you may need to repeat the remedy frequently because the 'energy' of the remedy may be used up by the body more quickly.

What if nothing has happened?
If you have taken 3-4 doses and there is no improvement, it may be a sign that a different remedy is needed. It is fine to try a new remedy if the first one did not help at all.

What if my symptoms change?
If symptoms change, then it is ok to change remedies (but remember some remedies, such as Pulsatilla, do have changeable symptoms as part of their picture).

When will I feel better?
The pace of the illness determines how quickly you can expect the remedies to work - for example, an individual with a migraine should respond quickly, whereas something like slow onset flu symptoms or chicken pox will take more time.

ALWAYS STOP TAKING REMEDIES ONCE YOU FEEL BETTER

The Homeopathic Law of the 'Minimum Dose' says you should take the smallest number of doses. The remedy only initiates self healing, so once that process has commenced, you can let the body do the rest. Always remember the innate wisdom of your body and what an incredible self healing machine it is.

 Please be sensible and use your judgement. If healing is not happening or it is a medical emergency, please seek help from an appropriate healthcare professional.

Acute Dosing

Can I take more than one remedy at the same time?
Ideally, just use one remedy at a time so that you can properly assess the reaction of the remedy. However, use your judgement - for example, in an emergency use Arnica and Aconite, alternating them in quick succession.

What potency?
30c is useful for most acute situations. 200c can be useful in extremely intense high energy situations, such as emergencies and childbirth. Lower potencies such as 6c or 12c may need repeating more frequently than high potencies. 30c is a brilliant universal potency. The remedy is much more important than the potency.

How many pills should I take?
Remember, homeopathy is energy medicine and very different from Western allopathic medicine. In homeopathy, it is the FREQUENCY of administering that counts as a dose; the pill is just a vessel for the energy of the substance, so it doesn't matter whether you give one, three or 10 pills when taken at the same time. Give just one pill to make the bottle/tube/packet of remedies last longer!

Is homeopathy safe and can it be used for babies or during pregnancy?
Yes, homeopathy is safe for newborns and during pregnancy and while breastfeeding. Remember these remedies only contain the energetic profile of the original substances. If you take the wrong remedy it simply will not work and as long as you do not continuously take it when not needed, it will do no harm.

How do I administer to a baby or someone who doesn't like the pills?
It is possible to 'water dose' remedies when administering to babies or those that don't like the pills. Simply dissolve one pill in water (or breast milk). The volume of water/milk that the remedy is dissolved in does not matter. One drop of that liquid then counts as one dose. You can keep the potentised liquid solution for 24-48 hours. This is a great way to also make a remedy last longer if you are down to your last pill and think you'll need multiple doses over a short period of time.

Acute Dosing

Can I eat or drink after taking the remedies?
Ideally, give 15 minutes away from food and drink and especially after cleaning teeth or drinking coffee.

How should I store my remedies?
Homeopathic remedies are energy medicine and should ideally be stored away from wifi. Keep away from strong smells and essential oils such as camphor, menthol and eucalyptus which can antidote the remedies.

Does it matter if I chew the remedy?
No, it does not matter. It will still work just fine if you chew the remedy.

Can I touch the remedies?
Remedies are delicate - touch as little as possible. Shake one pill into the lid and put straight into the mouth if possible. Alternatively, you can crush the remedy and put into water and sip - remember ONE SIP EQUALS ONE DOSE.

I felt so good on the remedy can I keep taking it?
Remember the Minimum Dose. Less is more with homeopathy! If you continually take a homeopathic remedy when it is not needed, you may experience a proving (highly unlikely in acute situations). Any symptoms produced during a proving resolve once the remedy is stopped.

What is a proving?
A proving is the homeopathic method of testing a substance on a healthy person. In a homeopathic proving, a homeopathic remedy is administered to healthy volunteers in order to produce the symptoms specific to that substance and thereby reveal its curative powers. If we continually take a homeopathic remedy when we are in a healthy state we risk proving the remedy. This is why we should only take homeopathic remedies when we have symptoms and only take the minimum dose. Even if remedies are proved, symptoms will stop as soon as you stop taking the remedy.

With gratitude and thanks to Dawn, Felix and Sara.

Other Books by Lisa Strbac

'The Homeopath in Your Hand - 77 Remedies & How to Select Them Using Homeopathy HEALS' by Lisa Strbac

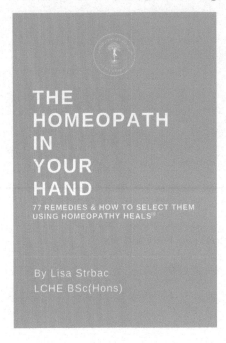

'The only book you'll ever need for home prescribing'

'I don't normally leave reviews but this book deserves one !! It's beautifully presented, easy to read and understand. A great book if you're new to homeopathy or already knowledgeable. I cannot recommend highly enough.'

'This book is AMAZING. So easy to follow, full beginners instructions, cheaper than booking a homeopathy appointment…Lisa you have smashed it. This book is going to fly into the world and change lives.'

'If you are new to or already have a knowledge of homeopathy, you don't want to miss out on this book! From homeopathy basics introduction and "how to" Heals method, to excellent summarization of most used 77 remedies & combination mixes, beautifully presented graphically, key symptoms and uses etc. This book is a must have! Very useful and small enough to take on travels!'

'Schuessler's Tissue Salts Rediscovered - The 21st Century Guide to Self-Healing' by Lisa Strbac

'Love your book! Great job. I have never seen a cell salt book that has so much useful information at a glance available for people of all knowledge levels. '

'Lisa has a gift to take overwhelming amounts of information and present it in a very reader friendly way without losing anything important. I love how this book has some history and the basis of what tissue salts are, very easy to go by key features of each salt, index of symptoms and even combinations and pregnancy sections. It has made my salt choosing for myself and my family more time efficient.'

'Love this book! Simple and so user friendly. Love the illustrations too which really bring the 12 tissue salts to life - it makes it easy to understand their essence and when they can be used.'

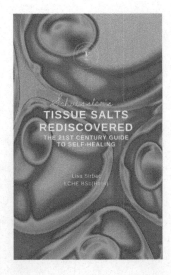

About Lisa Strbac
LCHE BSc(Hons)

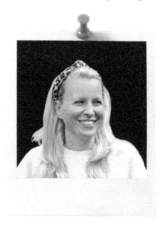

I am a certified Homeopath LCHE BSc(Hons), author of the bestselling books
'**The Homeopath in Your Hand'** and '**Schuessler's Tissue Salts
Rediscovered**' and host of the Raw Health Rebel podcast.

Previously a sceptic, but having exhausted all conventional approaches, my
journey towards holistic health started after witnessing the power of
homeopathy to heal my young daughter's chronic autoimmune condition. I
was so awestruck with homeopathy that I had to learn more, and, after 4
years of study and clinical practice, obtained my Homeopathy Licentiate. I
quickly left behind my corporate career and have been practising and
educating ever since.

My passion is to empower individuals to take responsibility for their own
health with the understanding that true health comes from within. My work
has evolved to teaching individuals how to use homeopathy at home. If every
individual had a basic homeopathy kit and knew how to use it, society's
mental and physical health would be transformed.

For more information on me and my courses you can connect with me at
www.lisastrbac.com.

Lisa Strbac

Made in the USA
Las Vegas, NV
28 November 2024

12831507R10125